What to Eat with IBD

What to Eat with IBD

✦

*A Comprehensive Nutrition and Recipe Guide for
Crohn's Disease and Ulcerative Colitis*

Tracie M. Dalessandro MS RD CDN

iUniverse, Inc.
New York Lincoln Shanghai

What to Eat with IBD
A Comprehensive Nutrition and Recipe Guide for Crohn's Disease and Ulcerative Colitis

iUniverse books may be ordered through booksellers or by contacting:

iUniverse
2021 Pine Lake Road, Suite 100
Lincoln, NE 68512
www.iuniverse.com
1-800-Authors (1-800-288-4677)

The information, ideas and suggestions in this book are not intended as a substitute for professional medical advice. Before following any suggestions contained in this book, you should first consult your personal physician.

Neither the author nor the publisher shall be liable or responsible for any loss or damage allegedly arising as a consequence of your use or application of any information or suggestions in this book.

ISBN-13: 978-0-595-39749-5 (pbk)
ISBN-13: 978-0-595-84156-1 (ebk)
ISBN-10: 0-595-39749-2 (pbk)
ISBN-10: 0-595-84156-2 (ebk)

Printed in the United States of America

This book is dedicated to my parents, whose love and support has been my guiding force in life. Thank you for educating me, loving me, and being my role models.

Contents

An inspirational message about living with IBD

Part I   Nutrition and IBD

An in-depth look at nutrition, food choices, and healing with IBD

A brief overview of Crohn's disease, ulcerative colitis, and IBS with
chronic diarrhea

Foods that heal and foods that hurt; how to maximize absorption,
choose the right foods for healing, and get enough protein and
nutrients

The prevalence of food-borne illness and how to avoid it; tips on
eating out and traveling with IBD, specific guidelines on keeping
food safe

Meals patterns for eating healthy with IBD, healthy snack ideas,
menus for everyday eating and shopping lists for easy planning

The importance of vitamins and minerals in IBD; essential
nutrients and recommended supplements, including forms and
brand names

Part II   *Nutrient-Rich Recipes*

Over 50 IBD-friendly recipes filled with nutrition. Each recipe includes a description of meal's nutritional qualities.

Acknowledgements

To my loving husband, Billy, who helped me make this book a reality, who spent hours editing my work, and who helped me believe I could accomplish this goal. Thank you for all your love and encouragement.

To my three beautiful children, Nina, William and Julia, who help me every day to be a stronger and better person.

Finally, to my four incredible sisters, who are there for me at every turn in the road. I love and admire all of you.

Preface
A Personal Story

The challenge of dealing with a chronic illness can change the course of one's life; it did for me.

At age nineteen, I was diagnosed with ulcerative proctitis, which progressed to ulcerative colitis and finally, at age thirty-one, Crohn's disease. Whatever one may call my elusive illness, the symptoms, both mental and physical, were the same—debilitating.

It was severe abdominal pain, diarrhea, and bleeding that brought me to the doctor in 1988. Once they told me what was causing these symptoms, I was relieved to finally have a name for this ailment that had consumed my life for over a year. Little did I know that it would only get worse from there.

Doctors described my disease as an inflammation of the large intestine and told me it would be a chronic condition. This is not something a nineteen-year-old wants to hear. Anyone who has the disease knows of the pain and embarrassment that goes along with it. I wanted it to go away, but I knew I had no choice.

At that point, doctors prescribed several medications for me and told me to reduce my stress. I asked about diet, considering the disease affected my intestines, but all they could tell me was that my diet would be based on trial and error. *How could something that so profoundly affects your gastrointestinal tract be based on trial and error?* After several more months of trying to heal and regain my strength, I knew there had to be another answer.

I decided to do my own research and spent months trying to uncover a diet that might help "cure" this disease. In my endeavors, I found my true passion. I realized the power of using diet in conjunction with traditional medicine to control my illness, rather than allowing it to control me.

Nutrition became the link between feeling sick and feeling well. I knew that my life's mission was to share this knowledge with others and help them to heal.

I went back to school to become a registered dietitian and to pursue a master's degree in nutrition. This gave me the credentials I needed to assist others in their healing process. Living with the disease gave me the experience of knowing the tribulations that go along with it. Since then, I have seen countless patients who suffer with IBD, all of whom have gained great rewards by improving their diet and learning which foods may trigger their symptoms. Working harmoniously with traditional and alternative medicine has helped many people get well and stay well.

To get well does not mean to "cure" this disease. It does, however, mean you can help heal the bowel and decrease the devastating symptoms of this illness. You can strive to educate and empower yourself physically, mentally, and spiritually. This book will guide you on the path to achieving optimal health with inflammatory bowel disease. It is the outcome of my trial and error.

Introduction
What This Book Is About

Healing, Believing, Following Through

It takes great courage, devotion, and strength to help your body recover from any chronic illness. I know firsthand what it takes—I have battled Crohn's disease for almost half my life.

The path can be long and arduous, but with determination you will get there. In the United States alone, over one million people suffer from inflammatory bowel disease. Unfortunately, there are many others who suffer in silence, not knowing what is causing their symptoms. There were many times I blamed my fatigue, diarrhea, and abdominal pain on food poisoning. It was not until these problems became chronic that I realized it was something else.

To live with this pain and do nothing about it is to accept a diminished existence in life. To take control of your health is to take responsibility for respecting and loving yourself.

I did not realize this until one day when I went to my gastroenterologist's office and he said something to me I will never forget. He said, "You have come to accept the pain and symptoms of this disease as a norm in your life. This is unacceptable." Living in fear and depression over a chronic illness does not have to be the "norm".

You can make a conscious effort to help your body heal and feel better. You must follow every turn in the road and persist even when you reach a dead end. Ask questions and insist on answers. Do your own research and educate yourself about your disease and all available treatments. Believe in your healing and work toward this goal. It will take time, energy, and faith to accomplish this task, but the rewards will be worth the effort.

This book will help you gain control over several major aspects of your recovery, and most importantly, it will teach you how to nourish your body and help your intestine heal using nutrition. The first chapter will give you a brief overview of Crohn's disease, ulcerative colitis, and irritable bowel syndrome. Subsequent chapters will discuss the principles of eating well with inflammatory bowel disease, food safety, meal planning and healthy snacks, and the importance of vitamins/minerals and the need to supplement. The second part of the book contains over fifty IBD-friendly recipes that are both nutritious and delicious.

The decision to take control of your health begins with good nutrition. You will be amazed at how some foods can make you feel horrible and others will make you feel well. I am not saying that you will never feel bad or have a flare-up. No one can predict the process of disease, and every case is different. What I am saying is that by following the dietary recommendations outlined in this book, you can minimize your symptoms of disease as well as the potential for flare-ups.

As I stated before, there is no cure for inflammatory bowel disease. There are, however, steps you can take to reduce the manifestations of disease.

The steps are as follows:

- Work with a gastroenterologist you can talk to and who helps you feel better emotionally and physically.

- Take your prescribed medications consistently.

- Follow a diet that promotes healing and rest for your intestines.

- Nourish your body with foods that contain a high amount of antioxidants, vitamins, and minerals to keep your body strong.

- Believe that you will get better.

- Find support in your endeavors through the Crohn's and Colitis Foundation.

I follow these steps with great conviction, and it has brought me very far in my recovery process. It is however, continual, and my inability to accept less out of life pushes me to strive for more.

Some Thoughts About Your Medication

As we embark on a discussion about healing, a word about your medication is necessary. Nutrition is one key component to being-well, but it should be used in conjunction with traditional medical care. Continuing any prescribed medicine is critical to bringing about remission and maintaining it. The nutrition principles and therapies outlined in this book are meant to be a complementary therapy to regular medical support.

I must also mention medicine and its relationship to nutrition. Certain medications make nutrition even more important to consider. Common medications that are given to IBD patients modulate or reduce the activity of the immune system. Medications like 6-MP, Imuran, methotrexate, and newer biologics like Remicade all reduce the immune response in the body. Considering that IBD is an autoimmune disease, it is reasonable to want to suppress the over-activity of the immune system. However, any therapy that reduces the immune system can compromise the body's ability to fight infection. This is where nutrition becomes imperative. Critical vitamins like A and C help the body to combat opportunistic infections and re-nourish the immune system. The goal is not to over stimulate the system but merely to enhance its ability to be well. Too often, IBD patients do not get enough of these micronutrients and feel depleted and fatigued. Restoring the body with nutrient-rich fruits and vegetables will help make a difference in overall health maintenance. The key is to take your medications, use nutrition to supply your body with vital nutrients, and understand that getting the body well is a process that involves many steps and great fervor.

PART I

Nutrition and IBD

As a dietitian, I have received many desperate phone calls from IBD patients. The calls usually sound something like this; "Please help me! I do not know **what to eat**. Everything I put in my mouth comes out as quickly as it went in. I can't leave my house and I can't eat anything."

As a patient myself, I always try to imagine what I would want to hear at that moment in time. My answer is always the same.

I would want someone to tell me that although things are out of control right now, it is temporary. I would want to hear that I will get better and that my bowel will calm down so that I could eat again. I would want to know that the fear and anxiety I am feeling is normal and that empowering myself through knowledge about treating my IBD will bring relief.

The truth is, this is the reality. In the throws of this illness we can feel out of control and desperate. However, things do get better and although we cannot always control what is happening to our bodies, we can control how we manage it.

Eating well, the right medication, and a good doctor to talk to will guide you to recovery. Inflammatory bowel disease is not a choice; it is a challenge that must be met with courage and conviction. Courage to let go of the fear that envelopes us when we are diagnosed with a chronic illness, and conviction to seek the best treatments possible and put our needs first.

Good nutrition is part of putting your needs first. It takes time and energy but is a necessary part of healing and being in control. Remember the old saying *"you are what you eat"* Its meaning in this context is profound. If you make healthier and better food choices, you will feel better. There has been an immense amount of research done on the benefits of nutrition in IBD. Read on to learn how you can incorporate these benefits to help reduce your symptoms and heal your body. If you make the right choices you will reap the rewards, and the rewards are many.

1

Who This Book Is Written For

When I was first diagnosed with inflammatory bowel disease, I looked for answers anywhere I could. I found several books that described the debilitating symptoms and complications that could arise with IBD (which consequently did not help my state of mind), but virtually nothing about diet.

I have written this book for those who wish to:

- Learn what foods help the bowel to heal and reduce the risk of inflammation and flare-ups

- Discover what foods help to re-nourish the body, improve their immune system, and promote energy and total health

- Discover the importance of proper digestion and nutrient absorption

- Learn recipes that have high nutrient value but do not cause distress on the bowel

- Empower themselves and take some control of their illness

I will not go into a deep discussion about pathophysiology (how the disease process affects the function of the intestine), symptoms, diagnosis, or complications of inflammatory bowel disease. There are many good books on the market that discuss these problems in detail. This book is meant to inspire and educate you about staying well, not teach what it means to be sick.

Those with Crohn's Disease

In brief, **Crohn's disease** is an inflammation that can affect the entire GI tract, but most often it strikes the lowest portion of the small intestine (*ileum*) and less often the large intestine. It is sometimes referred to as ileitis or Crohn's colitis, respectively. In 45% of cases, the disease will manifest itself in both the large and small intestine.

Crohn's disease can penetrate all the layers of the bowel and therefore can be more complicated than ulcerative colitis. Obstructions or strictures from inflammation and narrowing of the intestinal wall can make it difficult for food to pass by. The disease may be characterized by abdominal pain, diarrhea, weight loss, fatigue, growth failure, bleeding, fever, and general malaise.

These symptoms may be mild or severe depending upon activity of the disease. When Crohn's is active, one may say you are in a "flare." During the chronic phase of the disease, the symptoms may be quiescent and one may say you are in "remission." Remission must be achieved through medication and appropriate diet. If you are vigilant about both, you can be well for long periods of time.

Those with Ulcerative Colitis

In contrast to Crohn's disease, **ulcerative colitis** does not affect the entire GI tract. Only the large intestine or colon is involved, and the degree to which the disease is present varies. One may only have **proctitis,** which causes inflammation in the rectum, **distal colitis**, which affects the rectum and sigmoid colon, or **pan colitis**, which results in an inflammation of the entire large intestine. Ulcerative colitis does not affect the entire thickness of bowel, only the uppermost mucosal layers.

Symptoms in ulcerative colitis are similar to those in Crohn's disease, but bleeding and diarrhea may be more prominent in UC. Treatment options for both diseases are similar and rely on medication and dietary management.

Why are there special dietary needs?

With Crohn's disease, the entire GI tract may be affected; therefore, special attention must be paid to nutrition. Since Crohn's most often resides in the small intestine, malabsorption of nutrients is common. The small intestine is the body's main area of absorption for all macronutrients (protein, fat, and carbohydrate) and micronutrients (vitamins and minerals). When capacity is diminished, vital nutrients do not get into the bloodstream for delivery to body cells and organs. This can cause tremendous distress on the body.

Poor nutrition coupled with lack of appetite can lead to catastrophic nutrient deficiencies. When you add in diarrhea, fluid loss, and electrolyte loss, the results can be devastating. Severe weight loss, protein energy malnutrition, and vitamin and mineral imbalances result. Patients feel fatigued, weak, exhausted, and depressed.

Correcting these deficiencies and replacing fluids is a cornerstone in the nutritional treatment of Crohn's disease. Proper food choices and a diet that is rich in nourishing and nutrient-dense foods is the answer to staying well.

Nutritional needs in ulcerative colitis are similar to those in Crohn's disease; however, deficiencies may not be as severe. Since colitis affects only the large intestine, the small intestine functions well and absorptive capability is usually not diminished. I say "usually" because sometimes peristalsis (the rhythmic movement of food through the GI tract) is so rapid, and the diarrhea so severe, that the small intestine does not have the chance to absorb the nutrients from the food consumed. Blood loss in colitis may be more severe and iron deficiency anemia more common.

Similar to Crohn's disease, electrolyte, fluid, and nutrient deficiencies occur. The severity of these problems depends on the degree of disease activity and extent of colon that is involved. If someone has ten bowel movements per day, it is likely that they will feel quite weak and sick in comparison to a person who only has three or four bowel movements.

Nutritional Goals for Inflammatory Bowel Disease

In terms of the nutritional treatment of Crohn's disease and ulcerative colitis, I will not differentiate between the two. The goals in both diseases are the same:

Reduce inflammation and bowel irritation through nutritionally rich foods that nourish and heal the bowel. This will allow for restoration of nutrition status, bowel rest, and overall improved health.

The following principles apply to this goal:

1. Eat fruits and vegetables that soothe the bowel and avoid those that irritate.

2. Choose grains and breads rich in soluble fiber and avoid those with high contents of insoluble fiber.

3. Choose oily fish over meat as often as possible to replenish essential oils that coat the bowel and reduce inflammation.

4. Avoid an excess of dairy, which promotes mucous production, and use appropriate calcium substitutes.

5. Avoid fried, processed, and cured foods, which irritate the bowel and can cause diarrhea.

6. Cook healthy, nutrient-rich foods that are easily digested and absorbed.

7. Replace losses with the proper supplements in the amounts and forms necessary.

In the next chapter, I will discuss these principles individually and go into depth on how to apply them.

Those with Irritable Bowel Syndrome (IBS) Whose Chief Symptom Is Diarrhea

IBD distinguishes itself from IBS in several different ways. Foremost, in IBS there are no clinical or diagnostic changes in the bowel—it appears "normal" upon colonoscopy and biopsy. There is, however, the presentation of symptoms ranging from diarrhea to constipation, bloating, pain, and spastic colon. Although these symptoms may be severe and mimic those of IBD, there is no bleeding or inflammation in the colon. The only manifestation of disease is symptomatic.

There have been several books written for IBS sufferers and many of them say the IBS "diet" is also successful for Crohn's and colitis patients. This is not truly the case. IBS sufferers sometimes have more constipation than diarrhea, and a high fiber diet is necessary.

With IBD a high-fiber diet can cause excess damage to the bowel when inflammation and ulceration is severe.

One must look at the two disorders symptomatically in order to find the right diet. *IBS sufferers whose chief complaint is diarrhea can find relief if they follow the recommendations outlined in this book. The goal is to reduce the consumption of distressing foods, which in turn will reduce the incidence of spastic colon and watery stool.* Be wary of books that prescribe a high fiber diet for all IBS patients. Many advocate eating raw vegetables, nuts, high fiber grains and seeds. This advice could be devastating for IBD patients and could cause great distress for IBS patients who have a lot of diarrhea.

The Digestive Process: An Overview

Before we can move on, it is necessary to understand the inner workings of the digestive process. Familiarize yourself with the functions of both the small and large intestine so you can understand how your disease affects your body. The different areas of the GI tract have various "jobs" that make each very specific in function. If you know where your disease is located in the bowel, you will be able to see what macro and micro-nutrients might be of issue to you.

MAJOR ABSORPTIVE SITES IN THE GI TRACT

SMALL INTESTINE

DUODENUM-
Iron, Calcium,
and Magnesium

JEJUNUM-
Carbohydrates
(Sugars),
B Vitimans,
Vitamin C and
Protein
(Amino Acids)

ILEUM-
Vitamins A,D, E,K,
Fat, Bile Salts,
B12, and
some minerals

**LARGE
INTESTINE**

COLON-
Potassium,
Sodium, Water,
(Formation
of Vitamin K)

2

The Eight Principles of Eating Well with Inflammatory Bowel Disease

Whenever I see a client for the first time, I ask him or her to visualize the following situation: imagine having an open wound on your hand. Look at it. See the red, swollen, inflamed, bleeding tissue. Now imagine rubbing that wound with a nutty grain bread or raw vegetables, tough apple skins, or popcorn. Do you think that would help that wound to heal? Of course not—it would be like rubbing sandpaper on an open sore. Now imagine that wound in your intestines. What would you choose to rub on there?

In this chapter, I will discuss the "eight principles" for eating well with IBD. These principles detail many of the foods that help nourish and heal the body as well as those detrimental to your healing process. They should serve as a guide in terms of planning your diet and meal patterns. "Planning" is the key term here, because those with IBD need to think critically about what they choose to eat. If you fail to plan, chances are your diet will be lacking essential nutrition that you need to stay healthy. Use the "principals of eating well" to guide your food choices and take these three steps to apply the knowledge you gain:

1. *Have a plan for meals.* Make sure you understand the foods that help and harm you and plan your meals accordingly. Try not to make last-minute decisions when it comes to meal choices. If you do this, you will often end up eating fast foods.

2. ***Make lists for shopping.*** Use the principles outlined to make a food shopping list. If the appropriate foods are at your disposal, it will be easy for you to make good meal choices.

3. ***Set goals for nutrition.*** Study the principles outlined so you truly understand the value of each statement. Good nutrition does not come easy. You must apply constant effort to maintain a high-quality diet. It is not always easy for an IBD patient to do this, but if you understand what you can tolerate, you will be well on your way to better health.

In subsequent chapters, I will discuss more about meal planning, food safety, and nutritional supplements, all of which fall under the heading of "how to eat" with IBD. The principles outlined in this chapter cover "what to eat." Extensive research and experience are the basis for each topic that I will cover.

Criteria for Food Choices

Before embarking on a discussion about foods that heal and foods that hurt, you must understand the criteria for placing food in either group. The main reason that some foods are acceptable to eat and others not is fiber. Some fibers are just too difficult for an inflamed bowel to digest. Severe irritation and diarrhea can be caused by ingesting a food that is too rough or raw. This is especially true when inflammation is severe and narrowing of the gut is present.

I, as well as many of my patients, have found great relief during periods of exacerbation by being mindful of food choices. Some people tolerate certain foods better than others. However, the lists included in the principles outlined identify the most commonly irritating foods. You may choose to be more liberal with your choices once your inflammation has subsided; however, you should always consider what you are about to learn about fiber.

There Are Two Kinds of Fiber

Soluble Fiber

Soluble fiber can have tremendous benefits for patients with IBD. Quite simply, soluble fiber is "soluble in water," which means it has a great capacity for absorbing water in the GI tract. Soluble fiber forms a gel-like consistency in the gut when it moves through the system. This is beneficial for patients with diarrhea, because the absorption of water in the GI tract helps to slow the movement of food in the intestine. The outcome of slowing food in the intestine is increased absorption of nutrients and the lessening of diarrhea. Pectins and gums are two examples of soluble fiber with tremendous water-holding capacity.

Insoluble Fiber

Insoluble fiber is not soluble in water, which means that it actually draws water into the GI tract and makes the contents move more quickly through the system. In essence, it has the reverse effect of the soluble fibers. Insoluble fibers include cellulose and lignin and have poor water-holding capacity. Insoluble fiber does not form a gel with waste products in the gut but rather increases the bulk of waste and hastens transit time in the intestines. The outcome of such bulking and drawing in of water into the gut is diarrhea and irritation of the GI tract.

Now that you understand the basic differences between soluble and insoluble fibers, the question is "How do I get more soluble fiber into my diet while avoiding the less desirable insoluble fiber?" Unfortunately, the answer to that question is a bit difficult. In nature, fibers reside together, meaning that foods which contain soluble fiber also have insoluble fiber. Most fruits, vegetables, and grains have a combination of the two fibers. It is important to avoid foods that contain high amounts of insoluble fiber and eat more foods with soluble fiber.

Soluble fiber generally resides on the "inside" of food, whereas insoluble fiber exists on the "outside." A good example is an apple. The skin of an apple is insoluble and the inside is soluble. If I were to put the skin in water, it would not absorb it. However, if I take the inside of the apple, add water, and heat it, the apple becomes applesauce. Peas are another example of the soluble/insoluble combination. The outside skin of a pea is insoluble and the interior is soluble. Unfortunately, with peas, you cannot separate the fibers, and therefore peas are not recommended.

Considering all of the information you have learned about *soluble* and *insoluble* fibers, you will now be able to fully grasp how certain foods fit into the principles that follow.

The Principles

1. *Choose breads, cereals, and grains that soothe the bowel and avoid those that irritate it.*

Breads grains and cereals are often a large part of our diets. Making the right choices when it comes to these foods is an important part of helping your gut to heal. Making the wrong choices can be very detrimental to an intestine that is already inflamed. The right choices will provide nourishment and minimize symptoms, especially bleeding and diarrhea. If you recall the scenario at the start of the chapter, you will remember that extremely grainy, hard wheat products can cause increased irritation and do more harm than good.

Let's start our discussion about breads, grains, and cereals by applying the knowledge we have gained about fiber. Most whole-wheat and bran products contain high concentrations of insoluble fiber, whereas more highly processed breads and grains have the grain and bran removed. Any cereal or bread products containing a high amount of insoluble fiber should be avoided when inflammation is present. These include many whole-wheat products and highly seeded breads. Oats and oatmeal contain high concentrations of soluble fiber and are generally considered safe to eat. In choosing your grains, which include cereal, rice, pasta, bread, and crackers, keep these rules in mind:

• Avoid all grains with seeds, nuts, and high amounts of whole grains.

- Avoid whole-grain wheat and whole bran products, which are filled with insoluble fiber.

- Eat foods with oats because of the high content of soluble fiber.

- Eat grains that are more highly processed and finely milled.

As a dietitian, I find it difficult to recommend foods that are highly processed and low in whole grains. However, as an IBD patient, I know through experience that certain grains are extremely irritating to the gut and can cause severe diarrhea and malabsorption. It is unfortunate that some of the healthiest foods are not suitable for Crohn's and colitis patients, especially when it comes to grains. Be careful to make the right choices. Sometimes the healthiest choice is not the best choice when allowing your gut to heal.

Here are some examples of good selections:

Breads that Heal

Breads		Cereal
white	*Pasta*	Cheerios®
potato	white	Rice Krispies®
oatmeal (soft)		Rice Chex®
rye without seeds	*Crackers*	Kix®
sourdough	saltines	Life®
	Ritz®	Quaker Oatmeal Squares®
Rice	Keebler® townhouse	puffed rice
white rice	rice crackers any without whole grains	very soft cooked
instant brown rice	water crackers	oatmeal (great choice)
Arborio (short-grain white rice)		cream of rice

You may have noticed that on my list I did not include highly processed cereals that are high in sugar (such as Froot Loops® or Captain Crunch®). The reason they are not included is that I do not advocate eating a lot of high sugar content foods (above 6 grams of sugar per serving). While these selections will not harm you, sugar is a less desirable addition to food.

Breads that Hurt

Breads

Breads	Cereal	Pasta
Whole wheat	All-Bran®	whole wheat
rye with seeds	Shredded Wheat®	
any with whole grains	any with dried fruit/nuts	**Crackers**
any with nuts or seeds	Fiber One®	Trisket®
7-grain	Raisin Bran®	tortillas
12-grain	Wheeties®	multigrain
bran	Bran Flakes®	any with seeds
	Great Grains®	cracked wheat
Rice	Granola	
Whole grain brown	Grape Nuts®	
Wild rice		

2. *Always peel your fruits and choose fruits that heal.*

Fruit is an indispensable part of the diet. Fruit helps to nourish the body with a host of antioxidants, such as vitamins A and C, as well as critical electrolytes like potassium and sodium. Many people with IBD do not eat enough fruit because they fear it will worsen their symptoms when in fact, choosing the right fruit will help you avoid unnecessary pain and diarrhea.

When IBD is at its worst, the right fruits can provide incredible nourishment and essential nutrition that is easy to digest. There are many fruits that contain more nutrition than common vegetables. For example, cantaloupe, which can be easily added to a high-protein shake, contains the following nutrient content:

1 cup cubed cantaloupe:

- 62 calories
- 14.8 grams of carbohydrate
- 0 grams of fat or protein
- 547 mg of potassium
- 5,706 IU of vitamin A
- 75 mg of vitamin C

So, what exactly does the above nutritional information mean? Well, if you examine the daily requirements for common nutrients, you will find the Dietary Reference Intakes, a recommended level of nutrients established by the government, estimates our needs for these nutrients, to be the following:

- 5000 IU of vitamin A per day
- 60–75 mg of vitamin C per day

That means by consuming one cup of cantaloupe, you can meet your daily requirement for these vitamins.

All fruit should be peeled, especially apple, which has an extremely tough, fibrous skin. As discussed earlier in the section about fiber, the skin of fruits contains "insoluble fiber," which is very difficult for people with IBD to digest. These skins can cause severe irritation, bloating, and diarrhea. However, some individuals can tolerate some fruit skins. Skins on peaches and nectarines are not as tough and coarse as an apple skin and contain less insoluble fiber. These fruit skins may be tolerated, but only if diarrhea is not severe and acute. Soft fleshy fruits like mango, papaya, and melons (which are always peeled anyway) are very high in nutritive value and are well tolerated.

One final word about fruit: all berries (e.g., blueberries, raspberries, strawberries) should be avoided due to the seeds. The seeds, though tiny to the eye, are a major irritant to the bowel. Dried fruit is also unacceptable because of the excess skin around it.

Fruits that Heal (peeled)

apple, cooked	mango
apple, peeled (if no acute diarrhea)	nectarine
applesauce	papaya
apricot	peach
avocado	pear (cooked is best)
banana	pineapple
cantaloupe	plum
casaba melon	watermelon
honeydew	

Fruits that Hurt

blackberries	currents
blueberries	dates
cherries	figs
cranberries	grapefruit
grapes	raisins
kiwi fruit	raspberries
orange (due to membranes)	strawberries
pomegranate	tangerine
prunes	

3. *Always cook your vegetables and choose vegetables that heal.*

Just as fruit is a critical part of the diet, so are vegetables. Fruits and vegetables are the main source of certain vitamins and carotenoids in our diets. Limiting or avoiding these nutrients is detrimental to our overall health and is unnecessary as long as you know which vegetables to eat, which to avoid, and how to properly prepare and cook those vegetables.

Our bodies need vegetables to deliver an abundance of nutrients to our systems. Vegetables supply us with very concentrated amounts of vitamins A and C, as well as various phytochemicals that enhance and protect the body from disease. Although many of the beneficial compounds in vegetables are still being researched and discovered, what we do know is that substances like lycopene, flavanoids, and glutathione can help reduce our risk of cancer and chronic disease. Some of the greatest sources of those compounds are found in fruits and vegetables.

Vegetables are a necessary part of everyone's diet, especially those with malabsorption diseases. Those of us with diseases affecting the bowel actually need extra nutrients to help the body heal. I cannot tell you the amount of times I have looked at the diet of an IBD patient to see that it consisted solely of carbohydrate and protein. Understandably, IBD patients have a great fear of eating vegetables. However that fear must be tackled and overcome in order to change the quality of the diet and afford the body the nutrition it needs to heal. No diet can be complete without the inclusion of vegetables.

Following these steps will help to add vegetables back to the diet as well as minimize any symptoms of bowel distress.

- Always cook vegetables well

- Never eat raw vegetables with the exception of lettuce

- Avoid all vegetables with seeds

- Peel vegetables when appropriate

- Eat fresh when possible

• Be wary of gassy vegetables (see list)

Once again I will divide vegetables into two categories, those that heal and those that hurt. The criteria once again will be based on the fibrous content of the food. Remember that cooking changes the fiber matrix of food, making some vegetable acceptable when cooked and unacceptable raw.

A few vegetables that are on the heal list may cause distress due to the vegetables' tendency to cause gas. These include many of the cruciferous vegetables like broccoli and cauliflower. Cruciferous vegetables will not harm the bowel (when well cooked) but do cause bloating and distress in some people. Use trial and error in eating these choices.

Vegetables that Cause Gas

beans	garlic
broccoli	kohlrabi
Brussels sprouts	onions
cabbage	peppers
cauliflower	radishes
celery	turnips
eggplant	

Vegetables that Heal

acorn squash	lettuce (Bibb or Boston is best)
arugula	parsnips
asparagus	peppers, roasted without skin
broccoli (very soft)	parsnips
butternut squash	potatoes
carrots	pumpkin
cauliflower (very soft)	spaghetti squash

collard greens (very soft)	spinach
endive	sweet potato
kale (very soft)	tomato, without seeds
mushrooms	yam

Vegetables that Hurt

alfalfa sprouts	cucumber
bamboo shoots	eggplant
beans (all varieties)	garlic (for flavor is okay)
beets	onion (for flavor is okay)
beet greens	peas
Brussels sprouts	radishes
cabbage	sauerkraut
celery	string beans
corn	zucchini

As you may have noticed, many of the vegetables on the "hurt" list have *seeds* and *skins* that cannot be removed. Additionally, vegetables like cabbage and string beans have tough fibers that cannot be broken down enough by cooking and therefore should be avoided. Onion and garlic are good flavoring agents but should not be eaten in whole pieces. Lettuce, which is on the "heal" list, must be used with caution, especially when diarrhea is profuse. During an acute flare, I try to avoid any raw vegetables. All other greens, like kale and spinach, must be very well cooked.

4. *Choose foods with high nutrient density and avoid fast foods.*

Unfortunately, it is quite easy to choose foods that are quick to eat and have little nutritional value. As a society, we have encouraged the growth of major fast food chains that provide food that is less than adequate for the general population, and especially for people with IBD.

When you choose high quality, nutritious foods, you give your body the calories it needs as well as important vitamins and minerals it craves for health. Since many people with IBD suffer appetite loss, choosing foods that provide good nutrition in a small volume becomes a challenging task. If we bombard our bodies with foods that are low in nutrients and high in fat and sodium, we are wasting valuable space within the GI tract and are filling ourselves with poor quality food. Worse than that, the excess fat content in fast foods is difficult for your wounded GI tract to digest and leads to poor absorption. When fat absorption is incomplete, gas, bloating, and diarrhea are the outcome. This is especially true for people who have Crohn's disease in the small intestine or and those who have had much of the small bowel resected.

Avoid high-fat meals that cause malabsorption. Fried foods are especially culpable when it comes to causing diarrhea and pain. Avoid fried foods at all costs and be wary of heavily fat-laden meals, such as Chinese food, and fried Italian foods, such as chicken Parmesan. Spend more time preparing your own food, and when you go out choose foods that are baked, broiled, grilled (not charred), and sautéed. You will be quite surprised at the difference in how your body reacts and how your symptoms improve when you start making better food choices.

5. *Choose high-quality lean protein and avoid high-fat protein sources.*

Protein is a critical component of everyone's diet, but especially the IBD patient. Many research papers have been written about the problems that arise due to a lack of protein.

Protein deficiency among IBD sufferers may occur for two reasons: 1) chronic malabsorption and diarrhea, and 2) inadequate intake. Children with IBD are at the greatest risk when it comes to protein deficiency. When the body is in negative protein balance, it can cause severe growth failure, tissue wasting, muscle weakness, and poor immune function. Often, the initial diagnosis for Crohn's disease is identified among children because of a failure to thrive.

The IBD patient must not overlook high-quality low-fat proteins and should recognize them as necessary for proper growth and development. The body relies on protein for several critical functions, including

- Formation of hormones and enzymes

- Building and maintaining of body tissues

- Transport of vitamins and minerals

- Growth and repair

Proteins include the following kinds of food:

Complete proteins
fish
meat
poultry
eggs

Incomplete proteins
legumes
soy-based products
dairy
grains

The quality of ingested protein varies with each food. Animal proteins, such as meat, fish, and eggs, contain all essential amino acids that the body needs; therefore, they are "complete" proteins. Eggs are especially beneficial because they are inexpensive, easy to prepare, and rich in B vitamins and iron. Non-animal sources of protein (the "incomplete proteins") must be combined in order to get all the amino acids the body requires. For example, rice must be combined with beans, and peanut butter must be combined with wheat bread to make them complete proteins. The problem with this scenario is that IBD patients often cannot tolerate beans and wheat bread.

The best source of high-quality lean protein is fish. Fish also has the added benefit of essential fatty acids that help to suppress the body's inflammatory response. Recent research in Japan, Italy, and the U.S. has proven that people with inflammatory bowel disease have abnormal essential fatty acid profiles, which interferes with the renewal and formation of new cells in the gut. The suggestion, therefore, is to add more omega-3 and omega-6 fatty acids, which help heal the gut and squelch inflammation.

Other great sources of lean protein include
white-meat chicken
white-meat turkey
pork tenderloin
center-cut pork chops

Less desirable protein sources would include foods like
hot dogs
high-fat lunchmeat (salami, bologna)
high-fat ground beef
highly marbleized cuts of beef
bacon
sausage
meat with skin
ribs

Low-fat dairy and legumes, like soy and nuts (smooth peanut butter), are also good sources of protein. However, they are not complete proteins, meaning they do not contain all the essential amino acids that the body needs.

6. *Choose calcium-rich foods three to four times per day and supplement when necessary.*

Calcium is of great importance to everyone, but especially Crohn's and colitis patients. Osteoporosis is one of the most prevalent diseases that can be prevented through the appropriate intake of calcium. IBD patients are at greater risk than normal for osteoporosis due to chronic malabsorption, poor intake of dairy, and medications that deplete calcium from bones.

Osteoporosis is the clinical term for decreased bone density and brittle bones. It often leads to recurrent fractures and crippling deformities that are irreversible. The appropriate intake of calcium, vitamin D and vitamin A early in life is critical to the optimal deposition of calcium in bones. Bone growth and peak bone-mass development occurs only up until about the age of forty. Bone degradation (or resorption) exceeds formation from age forty on, therefore, it is critical to deposit enough calcium into bones early in life.

Calcium content in the blood is not an indicator of osteoporosis. The most effective indicator is a bone density test, which should be done on a regular basis to assess risk. There are currently several medications that help prevent osteoporosis, and early detection of the disease is critical to preventing further bone loss.

Postmenopausal females are at even greater risk due to hormone changes that make calcium absorption more difficult for the body. It is imperative for these patients to be fully evaluated for osteoporosis. Weight-bearing exercise along with good calcium intake and possibly medication are the answers to warding off this preventable disease.

Getting the appropriate amount of calcium rich foods is not always easy for IBD patients. I recommend 1200–1500 mg per day of this mineral, and even more if you are taking steroids. How do you get that much calcium? Eat at least three serving of calcium-rich foods per day and take a supplement for extra protection.

Calcium-rich food for IBD patients
(Each provides approximately 300 mg of calcium)
calcium-fortified soy milk (1 cup)
lactose-free milk (1 cup)
yogurt without added milk solids (1 cup)
aged cheese, if tolerated (1 oz)
soy protein powders with added calcium (1 scoop)

calcium-fortified orange juice without pulp (1 cup)
canned salmon or sardines (3 oz)

These foods are some of the highest calcium content foods. You will notice that dairy products dominate the list. That is because they are the best source of calcium. In addition, dairy is fortified with vitamins A and D, which help the body absorb the calcium it takes in. Unfortunately, many patients with IBD have to avoid milk because it is poorly tolerated and can cause excess mucus production. In this case, drink soy milk at least once a day to obtain a good amount of calcium.

You may be wondering why greens like spinach, kale, broccoli, and collards are not on my list. These vegetable sources of calcium have great nutritional value, but they are not the "best" sources of calcium, nor are they the most absorbable sources due to their content of oxalic acid. Oxalic acid binds to calcium and makes it less available to the body. You must concentrate on getting at least three servings of the "300 mg group" calcium foods and add greens and supplements for good measure.

7. Get enough fluids and calories throughout the day.

Fluids

The average person should ingest about 64 oz of water per day, or about eight glasses. *When diarrhea is present replacing those losses is even more imperative, and at least ten glasses of fluid should be consumed per day.*

Fluid in the form of water is best. However, when there are severe electrolyte losses from the gut (such as sodium and potassium), sports drinks diluted with water are acceptable. There are several products on the market, including Gatorade®, Powerade®, and Vitamin Water®, as well as the newer electrolyte waters. Another alternative is to mix a little orange juice in water. Orange juice has 400 mg of potassium in 8 oz, as well as folate, calcium, and vitamin C.

I recommend diluting drinks with water so that the concentration of sugar is not so high. Re-hydrating the body is necessary, but you need not consume excessive amounts of sugar.

Calories

Getting enough calories is sometimes a challenging task for IBD patients. Appetite loss can be a major symptom of disease, and fear of eating exacerbates this problem. I have seen many clients clearly avoid eating during the day for fear of stimulating the GI tract and having an "attack." This common fear leads to an energy deficit that causes depletion of body stores of protein and calories.

This protein-energy malnutrition is a common finding in IBD patients and must be countered by insuring that adequate caloric intake is measured. Beyond the poor appetite and patient restriction of food issues, the body's need for calories during times of stress (i.e., inflammation) is increased. Tissue breakdown and healing is a continuous process, and energy and protein needs become greater. If you have ever heard the saying "Feed a fever," you now understand why. The body uses calories and protein for healing. It raises its temperature to rid the body of infection, and when this occurs, the metabolic needs for energy increase. You must meet that demand, or the deficit will result in tissue wasting and weight loss.

In IBD, the need for extra calories depends on losses and inflammation. If there is significant weight loss, fevers, and inflammation, the need will be much greater than if weight is stable and someone is not actively in a flare. Use this simple calculation to determine caloric needs for times of stress and times of being well overall.

- *Caloric needs for stress (inflammation, fevers, diarrhea)*
  40–50 calories per kg body weight (1 pound equals 2.2 kilograms)

- *Caloric needs for wellness*
  35 calories per kg body weight

A typical calculation for someone who is in a flare would look like this:

Body weight = 150 pounds
↓
150 divided by 2.2 = 68 kg
↓

68 kg x 40 calories = 2720 calories per day

Getting about 2500–2700 calories would be adequate to meet metabolic needs; however, this is still a challenge for IBD patients. In the next chapter, I will detail the foods that are acceptable to eat. I will also cover a sample menu and how to add high calories to your diet.

8. *Maximize absorption*

The first part of digestion actually occurs in the mouth, when enzymes such as amylase start braking down food that has been masticated by chewing. Mastication is a critical aspect of digestion, because it allows for the proper absorption of food. When food is broken down into smaller particles, its passage through the GI tract is easier because the GI tract has less work to do. The better food is chewed, the easier it is on your entire digestive process. Follow these guidelines when eating:

• Eat in a relaxed atmosphere and try not to eat on the run.

• Chew food well before swallowing to allow for proper digestion.

• Eat slowly without gulping and swallowing air.

It is not uncommon for people with IBD to be put on "elemental" or liquid diets. The rational for this therapy is that it allows the bowel to rest and heal. When you chew your food well and eat slowly in a relaxed atmosphere, you are promoting similar benefits. Although this does not allow for total bowel rest, it does allow for easier absorption and digestion.

In Summary

Following these principles is critical in an acute flare situation. Acute flare means any inflammation in the GI tract, either upper or lower bowel. For some, a "flare up" may be less severe than for others. I have seen many patients who are in the bathroom over ten times a day with continual bleeding, fever, and pain. I have seen others who are only having two to three bowel movements per day but still have extreme discomfort from strictures or narrowing of the gut. There are also the occasional patients who present with constipation and vomiting because of inflammation in the upper part of the small intestine. My point is that every case of IBD is different and each person experiences things in his or her own way.

For this reason, it is imperative that you know your own body and your limitations. I have included in these "dietary principles" the most common foods detrimental in dealing with an acute inflammation situation. As your body heals and your intestine becomes less inflamed, you may be able to liberalize your diet to include foods with a little more fiber, such as the skin on a soft peach. That time would only come when there was very little diarrhea or discomfort in the intestine. However, always maintain caution when considering consuming nuts, seeds, popcorn, and raw vegetables. Take things day by day and know that your body can heal itself if given the time.

3

Food Safety

I will never forget the time I went to my husband's Christmas party at a nice restaurant in New York City. Dinner was served buffet style, and I ate off the buffet just like everyone else. When I tasted the food, I knew that it was not at the right temperature, but I decided to eat it anyway. Six hours later, I ended up in the emergency room with severe stomach cramping, diarrhea, and fever. Doctors were not quite sure at the time if it was the IBD flaring up or a bad case of food poisoning. The thing is, sometimes you just cannot tell the difference. Since I had been well for a long time and my intestines were not really inflamed, it was determined that I was suffering from "acute gastroenteritis," better known as food poisoning.

The Statistics

The Centers for Disease Control estimates that there are over 76 million cases of food-borne illness every year. That statistic translates into about one in four people getting sick from food on an annual basis. Of these reported cases, 325,000 people will have to be hospitalized and 5,000 deaths will occur in the United States alone. I mention these statistics to convey the importance of food safety.

The Causes

Food-borne illnesses are caused by pathogens in food, such as bacteria, parasites, and viruses. Many of these pathogens, such as e-coli and campy-lobacter jejuni, have been identified, but still many are unknown because they have yet to be determined. Of all food-borne pathogens, bacteria most commonly cause illness. These microorganisms can thrive and multiply rapidly when food is not handled or stored properly. Parasites in food can be ingested when food is not cooked properly (such as pork and fish), or they can be transmitted in unsanitary water. Viruses, such as Norwalk virus, are contracted through ingesting food or water contaminated with human waste. Raw shellfish is especially culpable in causing this virus in people when it is harvested from contaminated water. Any of these pathogens can lead to illnesses in humans that last from several days to several months. Although rare, there have even been cases reported where bacteria from food has led to chronic diseases.

The Susceptibility Factor

People who are most susceptible to contracting a food-borne illness are the very young, the very old, and those who are immunocomprimised. Underlying medical conditions such as certain diseases, pregnancy, and poor nutritional status can also increase the likelihood of getting sick from contaminated food. People who take antibiotics that disturb the natural flora in the intestine or people that take immunosuppressant drugs (like corticosteroids and 6-MP) are also at greater risk. As an IBD patient, you are more susceptible due to the intestinal disease and the fact that you may be receiving treatment with antibiotics or immune compromising drugs.

The Contraction Factor

Food-borne illness, whether it is bacterial, parasitic, or viral, is usually contracted because of poor food handling. Poor food handling methods include inadequate hand washing by food handlers, keeping food at unsafe temperatures that allows the growth of bacteria, incomplete cooking of potentially hazardous foods, cross-contamination of raw food with cooked food, and improper washing of fruits and vegetables. Food that is safe when it arrives at a food establishment or supermarket can quickly become contaminated if it is stored improperly or prepared in an unsafe manner. It is imperative that all food handlers, including those that prepare food at home, educate themselves about the risks of food-borne illness and how to prevent them.

IBD and Food-borne Illness

As you may see from these statistics, the foods you choose to consume and how those foods are prepared affect your individual risk for food-borne illness. In earlier chapters, we discussed "What to Eat with IBD," however, in order to stay well, you must also know how to keep foods safe and what foods to choose when eating out. Poor kitchen sanitation and food preparation can lead to food-borne illness, which can be devastating to IBD patients. It is important to recognize that making the right choices when traveling and dining out is an important part of keeping yourself healthy.

While the general population may have no problem consuming foods that are mishandled *slightly,* this is not true for the IBD patient. In the example I gave at the beginning of the chapter, I did not tell you one thing. I was the only one who ended up sick that night. No one else got food poisoning, because no one else was as susceptible as I was. The likelihood that we will contract a food-borne illness is greater. An IBD patient must be careful and make the right food choices; taking the time to eat safely is paramount to staying healthy.

In general, IBD patients are more susceptible to food-borne illness for three primary reasons. First, we have an imbalance of bacteria in the gut that more readily predisposes us to bacterial contamination. It has been postulated that the potentiation of the immune system in IBD is caused by a bacteria. Second, many medications, such as antibiotics, cause this imbalance to become more severe. Antibiotics are not selective when it comes to killing bacteria in our systems. They kill the good and the bad, leaving us depleted of the "friendly" bacteria that keep our bad gut flora in check. Third, many of the medications we take, such as prednisone and 6-MP, reduce the activity of the immune system, lessening our ability to fight off pathogens. When you combine all of these factors, the risk is even greater.

IBD and Eating Out

Have you ever gone into your local deli or coffee shop and seen the sandwiches on top of the counter just sitting there, uncovered, not refrigerated and exposed to the air? This is the perfect example of how to be exposed to food-borne illness. Food-borne illness is a disease or illness carried to human beings by or through food. It most often occurs due to poor food handling. This is a perfect example of poor handling!

IBD patients must be especially vigilant when it comes to eating at restaurants and fast-food establishments.[1] A case of food-borne illness can exacerbate an underlying disease such as Crohn's disease or ulcerative colitis, causing the worsening of symptoms. Food-borne illness can even mimic the symptoms of disease, confusing the diagnosis. I understand that we are often forced to eat out or to eat on the run. However, it is critical that you understand what to look for when eating at restaurants in order to keep yourself safe. Does the restaurant look well kept and clean? Is the food refrigerated properly and stored properly? Is there soap in the bathroom so employees can wash their hands? These may seem like simple questions, but they are important.

Fast-food restaurants and fine-dining establishments must be scrutinized equally. Remember my example in the beginning—the food that I got sick from came from a "good" restaurant. However, the hot buffet was not being kept at the right temperature, and enough bacteria multiplied in the food to make me sick.

Keep this information in mind when eating out.

1. High-protein foods are responsible for most food-borne illnesses. These include milk or milk products, eggs, meat, poultry, fish, shellfish, and soy-protein foods that have been improperly refrigerated or handled.

2. Unwashed vegetables, including lettuce, potatoes, and onions, can be sources of bacteria. Make sure they are clean before eating them.

3. Avoid all food that has not been properly refrigerated, especially meat sandwiches left out on counters, soups that have not been heated to

---

1. Bean and associates reported that approximately 80% of reported food-borne illness was contracted outside the home in restaurants and fast-food venues.

the correct temperature, and any other items that have been left out for display without the proper refrigeration.

4. Avoid eating mayonnaise products that have been left out, especially during warm months. Tuna salad is especially questionable when not prepared at home.

5. Avoid raw and undercooked fish such as sushi, sashimi, rare tuna, and salmon.

6. Avoid salad bars, which are often not cold enough to keep food safe and which are often contaminated with other foods and human contact.

7. Do not eat rare chopped meat or steak, which are susceptible to e-coli. Make sure that all meat consumed is well cooked.

8. Be wary of eating at buffets that contain food that has been re-heated, may be cross-contaminated, or has been around to long. Meats in sauces are a breeding ground for bacteria.

9. Do not consume unpasturized milk or milk products, such as certain soft cheeses.

Understand the Potential for Food-borne Illness at Home

When preparing food at home, use the preceding information as well as the following:

1. Wash hands thoroughly when cooking. Twenty seconds with soap and water is what it takes to get them clean.

2. Use separate cutting boards for meat, fish, and vegetables to avoid cross-contamination of foods.

3. Refrigerate foods promptly. Do not leave food out on the counter to cool. Cover it and refrigerate it.

4. Cook food thoroughly, especially meat and fish. Use a thermometer that tells you the internal temperature when necessary. Some meat thermometers even tell you which temperature your particular meat should be (for example, pork should be 165°F).

5. Thaw foods in the refrigerator. Many people leave food on the counter to thaw. The outside will then thaw faster than the inside, leaving it more vulnerable to bacteria.

6. Re-heat foods to 165°F.

7. Sanitize work surfaces after cooking. Use paper towels to wipe counters and put sponges in the dishwasher every night.

After learning all of this information, I still have patients ask me, "So, what are the best ways to eat on the run and still eat safe?"

1. Know the places in your area that are well managed and clean.

2. Don't choose food that has been left out. Always ask for food to be freshly prepared, such as a turkey wrap.

3. Make sure salad is clean and dressing is cold.

4. If you choose to eat hot food, make sure it is hot and do not accept room-temperature or even warm food.

5. Never feel bad about sending food back. If it is cold or does not smell or look right, go with your gut and send it back!

Eating food that has been contaminated or poorly handled can lead to an exacerbation of disease. Bacteria that form on improperly prepared or stored food, leading to food-borne illness, can aggravate an already inflamed gut. If you are careful in choosing your meals, you will be much better in the end. There will be times when making good choices is difficult, especially when traveling. I have ended up in a few emergency rooms on vacation. Preparing yourself for travel is important. Always know what to look for in terms of choosing safe food and bring food with you so you don't go hungry.

In Summary

It is not always easy to make the right choices when eating out or eating on the run. The critical aspect is to "think" about what you can eat and "observe" what is going on in the food establishment. Ask yourself if the food looks appealing and if service areas and clean and well maintained. Also, be sure to choose the right foods for you. Try not to eat off salad bars and hot food stations that have had food sitting out for long periods of time. If possible, choose something freshly prepared over food on a buffet. It is not that this kind of food is always contaminated; it is just that the likelihood is greater. Some well-kept fast food establishments have good sanitation practices, but many do not. Reflect upon the recommendations outlined in this chapter. It will hopefully prevent unnecessary bouts with food-borne illness.

Be sure to observe proper preparation and handling of food at home as well. Food-borne illnesses are not only contracted in restaurants; they can be caused by poor food handing at home. Follow the guidelines discussed and familiarize yourself with food-safety behaviors. Good sanitation is imperative in preventing unnecessary food-borne illness.

4

Planning Your Meals

As discussed briefly in earlier chapters, planning meals is critical to keeping yourself well when you have inflammatory bowel disease. I see so many patients who fail to plan their meals because they are too busy or too lazy. They end up eating breakfasts that are filled with sugary carbohydrates, lunches that consist of a deli sandwich, and fast-food dinners. This kind of eating pattern is unnecessary and unhealthful. The lack of planning leads to a diet insufficient in nutrients and quality.

The best way to be prepared to eat well is to make a shopping list at the beginning of the week. Use this list to plan healthy meals and have good-quality snacks at your disposal. Your shopping list should be a compilation of foods from each food group and should look something like this one.

Dairy

lactose-free milk

yogurt

soy milk

Protein foods

smooth nut butters

chicken breast

fresh fish

turkey breast

lean pork chops

Pantry items

chicken broth

soy protein powder

Fats

olive oil

canola oil

Breads and grains

white rice

oatmeal

oatmeal bread

potato bread

plain crackers

Vegetables

asparagus

butternut squash

spinach

carrots

broccoli

Fruit

cantaloupe

banana

applesauce

peach

papaya

mango

avocado

Having a Plan

Once you have the right foods at your disposal, knowing how to plan healthy meals is the next important step in the process of eating well. Since you are now well aware of the foods that may cause distress and the foods that will help your gut to heal, you can readily use those lists to create your healthy eating plan. If you have days when you really don't want to eat, concentrate on fluids.

Fluids

Fluids are often overlooked and are critical to maintaining proper electrolyte balance. Always drink plenty of water. During acute periods of diarrhea, it is helpful to replace lost electrolytes with sports drinks and vitamin waters. I also find there are some days when I may just have less of an appetite and would prefer to drink some of my meals. On these days, I concentrate on getting calories through high protein shakes made with soy protein powder and a whole banana (for potassium). Go to the recipe section of this book for other ideas on healthy shakes and use them when appetite loss is significant.

Snacks

In terms of planning healthy snacks, think about combining foods with different qualities. For example, combine protein with carbohydrate, and fruit with dairy. The reason for combining is to get vitamins and minerals from at least two food groups. When you eat from one food group, you do not get as much value from the meal. It will not hurt you not to combine; it is just healthier to do so. Here are some examples of quality snacks:

- Peanut butter with crackers

- Yogurt with cantaloupe

- Soy protein shakes with banana

- Skinless apple or banana with peanut butter

- Cheerios with lactose-free milk or soy with banana

- Applesauce with plain yogurt

All of these snacks are better choices than having just a bowl of pretzels or a few crackers.

Meals

When planning meals, it is important to look at the day as a whole and try to incorporate as many colorful foods as possible. In general, the deeper and more colorful your meals are, the healthier they are. Richly colored fruits and vegetables should be a priority in planning meals. Many IBD patients feel that a bagel and coffee is a safe and sufficient breakfast and that a turkey sandwich on white is a perfect lunch. If you look at those meals, visually you will find them very white and lacking the nutrition that the body needs. Dinner is probably then made up of roasted chicken and a baked potato. Again, safe, predictable foods are fine, but as a whole the meal is lacking critical nutrients.

Here is an example of a meal plan I would recommend to IBD patients:

Breakfast:	1–2 egg omelet with spinach 1 slice potato bread ½ banana 6 oz calcium fortified orange juice
Snack:	½ cup plain yogurt mixed with ½ cup natural applesauce
Lunch:	White meat turkey w/mayo 2 slices oatmeal bread ½ cantaloupe
Snack:	Healthy fruit/protein smoothie
Dinner:	Grilled salmon with honey/Dijon White rice cooked with herbs and broth Roasted or grilled asparagus Small salad with Bibb lettuce

You will notice in this eating plan that each meal has been planned with purpose. The National Institutes of Health now recommends nine servings of fruits and vegetables per day instead of five. That is a tall order, considering most Americans do not even eat three servings. You must make a conscious effort to plan meals that incorporate many nutrients, including fruits and vegetable, with a good amount of vitamins C and A, foods with calcium, protein, and good complex carbohydrates.

If we break down this menu, you will find the following:

- 9 servings of fruits and vegetables

- 3 servings of calcium-rich foods

- 3 servings of lean high-quality protein

- complex carbohydrate

You may be looking at this eating plan saying, "This is too difficult" or "It takes too much time." Perhaps this particular plan is not the most practical for you, but if you are creative, you can simplify this plan to meet *your* requirements. Your healthy breakfast may be as easy as boiling an egg and having it with a piece of fruit. You can even prepare that the night before to save time. Maybe breakfast is a slice of oatmeal bread with smooth peanut butter and a banana on top. This breakfast takes about three minutes to prepare and is well rounded, consisting of protein, carbohydrate, and fruit. These examples show you how to incorporate healthy eating into your life with a little planning. It is not as difficult as you think; it just takes a bit of effort. Use this chart to help you plan healthy meals.

There are four choices here for each meal:

Breakfast:	Well-cooked oatmeal with banana
	Homemade soy shake
	Soy or regular yogurt with cantaloupe
	Hard-boiled egg with oatmeal toast

Lunch:	Sliced chicken breast on potato bread with fruit salad
	Turkey burger on roll with cooked vegetable
	Grilled chicken sandwich with fruit
	Tuna sandwich on oatmeal bread with small salad
Dinner:	Swordfish with teriyaki glaze, rice, and asparagus
	Roasted chicken with herbs, skinless potato, and candied carrots
	Broiled center-cut pork chops with applesauce and butternut squash
	Vegetable soup with French bread and small salad

These are just a few ideas to get you started. Turn to the recipe section of the book for other great meal ideas and add snacks for extra nutrition and calories.

When you start eating this way, with the foods that help your body to heal, you will find that you feel much better and have more energy and stamina. Fueling your body with the appropriate vitamins and minerals is critical to overall health and healing.

Tips on Increasing the Caloric Content of the Diet

For many people with IBD, weight loss is a significant factor. When the disease is extremely active, people can lose many calories per day through diarrhea and increased metabolic needs. Fevers and inflammation cause stress on the body, leading to an increase in caloric expenditure.

When it is necessary to increase the caloric content of the diet without having an excessive volume of food, healthy fats are the best source of calories. As discussed in Chapter 2 our caloric needs can sometimes be greater than what we are able to consume due to poor appetite. Fats are the most highly concentrated form of calories, with 9 calories per gram of fat, or 100 calories per tablespoon (liquid fat).

Below are some suggestions for padding your diet with extra calories. These foods are concentrated sources of calories for the amount of food you need to consume, making it easy to get a lot out of a little.

- Peanut butter and other nut butters (smooth)

- Guacamole

- Hummus

- Heavy cream added to soups, cereal, or tea

- Flax seed oil added to protein shakes

- Butter on potatoes, on bread, and in hot cereal

All of these choices add 50–100 calories per tablespoon to the diet. They are all healthy fats with the exception of the heavy cream and butter. However, if there is no risk of cardiovascular disease, having some heavy cream or butter is acceptable.

In Summary

It is challenging to meet all of the suggestions for meal planning outlined in this chapter. However, if you plan, make shopping lists, and know how to incorporate the recommended foods into *your* healthy eating plan, you will be successful. Use these recommendations as a guide and you will be able to meet many of the nutrient requirements your body needs to be healthy. Many worthwhile things in life take time and energy. Learning to manage your disease with good nutrition and planning is one of them.

5

The Need for Vitamins and Minerals and When to Supplement

Why the Need Is So Great

Would you believe me if I told you that all people with Crohn's disease and ulcerative colitis absorb food perfectly well? Probably not. The truth is that many people with IBD do absorb food well, but most do not. There are many factors that affect how well your food is digested and absorbed. These factors include where your GI tract is inflamed, how severe your diarrhea is, and whether one has had a surgical resection. All of these conditions require special dietary management with specific concern taken to evaluate nutrient quality of the diet.

Inflammation in the Small Intestine

If you are affected with Crohn's disease in the small intestine, chances are that your absorption of micro and macronutrients will be compromised. The small intestine is the gastrointestinal tract's main area of absorption for all nutrients, including protein, fat, carbohydrate, vitamins, and minerals. Without proper functioning of this organ, malabsorption is common and inevitable. Fat-soluble vitamins, including A, D, E, and K, are especially difficult to replace when fat malabsorption is an issue. Replacement of these losses is vital in maintaining health of the immune system, mineralization of bone, and normal blood clotting.

Compounding this problem of malabsorption is poor intake due to appetite loss. Appetite loss may be precipitated by abdominal pain due to inflammation and possible strictures. For these reasons and many others, it is necessary to consume a diet that is high in nutrient density as well as one that is delivered to the intestine in a more absorbable easy-to-digest manner.

Inflammation in the Large Intestine

Severe inflammation in the large intestine occurs in ulcerative colitis and Crohn's colitis, leading to intractable diarrhea and dehydration. Again, with this condition, absorption of crucial dietary nutrients is compromised. The job of the large intestine is to absorb electrolytes and excess water, hold stool, and produce vitamin K. When this organ is not functioning properly, excess diarrhea can lead to nutrient deficiencies because food is passing too quickly through the GI tract, giving it little time to absorb necessary nutrients. In addition to that, bleeding can lead to iron deficiency, and fluid loss contributes to calcium and potassium imbalance. Once again, in this situation it is critical for IBD patients to consume a diet rich in nutrients, because inevitably some of your food will not be completely digested and absorbed due to the problem of rapid transit time through the gut.

Food as Medicine

When malabsorption to any degree is present due to intestinal loss of nutrients, one must compensate by improving the quantity and quality of the diet. As discussed in earlier chapters, one must concentrate on eating foods that help the gut heal and avoid eating foods that can be harmful. Besides eating foods that do not harm the GI tract further, it is important to consider the content of your diet in terms of vitamins and minerals. Many IBD patients avoid fruits and vegetables because they are afraid of causing a flare up. When these restrictive practices become consistent, the diet becomes deeply lacking in sufficient nutrients especially vital antioxidants, like vitamins A, C, and E, and carotenoids, like beta-carotene and lycopene. It has been shown that serum concentrations of beta-carotene, magnesium, selenium, and zinc were significantly lower in UC patients than in controls. In Crohn's disease, B12 and fat-soluble vitamins were compromised.

Here is a guide to help you see the functions of each critical nutrient that may be mal-absorbed in IBD.

Fat-Soluble Vitamins

Vitamin A—The first of four fat-soluble vitamins I will discuss is vitamin A, clinically known as retinol. Carotenoids like beta-carotene are known as pro-vitamin A because they can be utilized in the body to synthesize vitamin A as needed. High intake of beta-carotene is recommended to those at risk for vitamin A deficiency, because the body can make usable vitamin A from these pro-vitamins. Carotenoids are non-toxic and stored in the fat cells of the skin when there is abundance in the diet.

High doses of pre-formed vitamin A, such as in supplements, can be toxic and should be used cautiously. Eating beta-carotene–rich fruits and vegetables is safe and healthy. The RDA for vitamin A is 5000 IU (international units)/day. This fat-soluble vitamin is commonly mal-absorbed in patients with Crohn's disease, especially when the duodenum is affected. Higher intakes are necessary to prevent deficiency.

Body benefits: Vitamin A helps the body improve resistance to infections, supports growth and repair of tissue, helps maintain healthy skin, hair, and mucus membranes, and is critical for night vision. Beta-carotene is a powerful antioxidant that protects the body from free radical damage.

Best sources: Preformed vitamin A can be found in foods like liver, milk, and eggs. Pro-vitamin, A carotenoids like beta-carotene, can be found only in fruits and vegetables. Best sources include carrots, kale, sweet potato, spinach, cantaloupe, mango, and papaya.

Vitamin D—Calciferol is the clinical name for vitamin D and is the most active form in the body. It is the second of four fat-soluble vitamins. Vitamin D deficiency has been noted in those with inflammatory bowel disease, especially Crohn's disease, due to malabsorption of the vitamin within the small intestine. Any time there is a problem with fat malabsorption fat-soluble vitamins can be compromised. There is also evidence that chronic use of steroids, such as prednisone, can lead to problems with vitamin D metabolism, which further compromises body stores.

Vitamin D can be synthesized by the body by exposure to sunlight and is therefore often called the "sunshine vitamin." The RDA for vitamin D is 200 IU for adults and 400 IU for older adults; however, many experts are now recommending at least 600 IU due to vitamin D's importance in the prevention of bone disease.

Body benefits: Vitamin D is necessary for the formation of the skeleton and in maintaining homeostasis of minerals within bone. Vitamin D assists the body in the absorption of calcium and promotes mineralization of bone. Long-term deficiency of vitamin D can accelerate the onset of osteoporosis. Severe inadequacy of vitamin D can cause bones to become thin and brittle, leading to a disease called osteomalacia in adults or rickets in children. Although these diseases are generally not seen in the U.S. anymore due to the fortification of milk, it is not uncommon to see a deficiency among those who do not drink milk and have a problem with fat malabsorption.

Best sources: Food sources of vitamin D include fortified milk, eggs, butter, and margarine. Calcium supplements usually include vitamin D as well. The body is capable of synthesizing enough vitamin D with adequate exposure to sunlight (fifteen minutes three times per week). Many patients with IBD avoid milk products, therefore a calcium supplement that includes vitamin D should be taken, along with some responsible time in the sun.

Vitamin K—Vitamin K is the third of four fat-soluble vitamins, and as with other vitamins that require fat to be absorbed, vitamin K status can be compromised by people with fat malabsorption diseases. Forty to seventy percent of vitamin K is absorbed in the jejunum and ileum, the two last portions of the small intestine. In several authoritative studies, it was found that serum vitamin K levels were significantly reduced in IBD patients as compared to controls. This is probably a major contributing factor in the development of osteoporosis. Vitamin K is poorly absorbed by the large intestine; however, bacteria in the colon actually produce about half of the vitamin K we need. This, of course, only occurs in a healthy gut. The RDA for adults is 65–80 ug. per day.

Body benefits: Vitamin K is necessary for the formation of prothrombin, a protein involved in regulating of blood clotting. The second-most important role of vitamin K is its role as a cofactor in the production of osteocalcin, a protein essential for helping calcium bind to bone. Vitamin K is also responsible for the formation of at least five other proteins, found in plasma, bone, and the kidneys. Deficiency, however, is usually only noted by defective coagulation of blood.

Best sources: The best food sources of vitamin K include green leafy vegetables such as spinach, kale, and broccoli. Synthesis of vitamin K in the large intestine also provides a substantial amount of what our bodies require. A good intake of vitamin K–rich greens and a multivitamin that contains a supplemental dose is a good way to avoid deficiencies of this vitamin, especially for those patients with Crohn's disease that affects the small intestine.

Vitamin E—The last of the four fat-soluble vitamins is vitamin E. After doing much research on IBD and micronutrient deficiencies, I was unable to find significant evidence that this vitamin is compromised. Therefore, I will only mention a few facts. Vitamin E is a major antioxidant that helps to protect our body's tissues from damage. It also helps in the formation of red blood cells and in the body's use of vitamin K. The richest sources of vitamin E are common vegetable oils as well as green leafy vegetables.

Water-Soluble Vitamins

Vitamin C—Vitamin C, also known as ascorbic acid, is a water-soluble antioxidant. Deficiencies of vitamin C, noted as scurvy, are rarely seen in the United States except among infants fed only milk or among the elderly population who are fed limited diets. I mention this vitamin because among IBD patients, there is often a lack of fruit and vegetable intake, and most vitamin C–rich food (approximately 90%) comes from these sources. Vitamin C is non-toxic; however, excess intakes as a supplement can cause diarrhea. The RDA for vitamin C is 60 mg.

Body benefits: Vitamin C is responsible for the protection of body tissues from oxidation, as it is a major antioxidant. Antioxidants in general protect cells against free radicals. Free radicals are potentially damaging products of the body's metabolism that can cause cell damage leading to the development of cardiovascular disease and potentially cancer. Vitamin C is also critical for wound healing, formation of collagen, and appropriate immune responses. Vitamin C enhances the intestines ability to absorb iron by two-to fourfold.

Best sources: As stated before, the best sources for vitamin C are fruits and vegetables. The fruits and vegetables with the highest concentrations include red peppers, broccoli, kiwi, citrus, collard greens, spinach, tomatoes, and strawberries. Approximately 90% of vitamin C in our diets is found in these sources. Protein and dairy products are sometimes fortified, accounting for about 10% of our intake.

B Vitamins—The B vitamins include riboflavin, thiamin, vitamin B6, B12, and folate. Of all the B vitamins, I will discuss folate in the most depth. Deficiencies of B vitamins used to be common; however, with the fortification of grains and other foods, B vitamin deficiency has become rare in this country.

B12 must be considered separately among Crohn's disease patients whose inflammation exists in the ileum or among those who have had small intestine resections involving the ileum. In these cases, B12 is not absorbed even when taken as a supplement by mouth, because the body cannot uptake the vitamin due to ileal damage or loss. Dietary B12's main absorptive site is in the ileum with the aid of intrinsic factor. Intrinsic factor is a glycoprotein that is produced in the stomach but acts in the small intestine by binding to B12 and allowing the vitamin to be absorbed by the ileal mucosa. People with ileal issues must get injections of this vitamin to avoid the development of deficiencies, such as pernicious anemia.

Consuming a diet that has adequate amounts of protein, including chicken, beef, fish, liver, pork, and eggs, as well as fortified foods like cereal and grains, provides enough of the B vitamins to sustain health. Again, the exception is B12 among those with damage to the ileum.

A separate discussion about folate is warranted due to the critical nature of this B vitamin. Folate is also known as folacin and is a critical B vitamin. Folic acid is the supplemental form of the vitamin. Folate is necessary for nucleic acid synthesis (DNA), and a deficiency of this vitamin leads to impaired cell division and alterations in protein synthesis. This most often affects rapidly growing tissues. Folate is also necessary for proper red blood cell formation and the metabolism of fats, proteins, and carbohydrates. In recent years, many food items have been fortified with this vitamin due to evidence that it protects fetuses from neural tube defects. The recommended intake is currently 400 mcg, but if you ever examine the contents of a prenatal vitamin, you will find the level to be as high as 1 mg.

Body benefits: For IBD patients, folate is especially critical. Remember, folate is necessary for proper cell division, especially in rapidly growing tissues. When inflammation has damaged tissues they are constantly changing and repairing, cell division is a continuous process. *Research has found that folic acid can help to keep those rapidly dividing cells "normal" and reduces the risk of dysplasia (abnormal cells), or cancer.* Many research articles have examined the relationship between folic acid supplementation and the decreased risk for dysplasia and cancer, especially in ulcerative colitis patients. The decrease in risk may be as high as 46% in those supplemented with folic acid. A detailed list within the reference section of this book will guide you toward the literature. Evidence for the benefits of taking extra folate is compelling and it continues to be studied as a means of chemoprevention in IBD patients. Medications, like sulfasalazine also compete with folate absorption in the body; therefore, a supplement is necessary to maintain normal body processes.

Best sources: The best sources of folate in the diet is leafy green vegetables, like spinach, kale, and romaine lettuce, some fruits, liver, legumes, and yeast. It should be noted that as much as 50% of folate can be destroyed in everyday preparation and storage.

Minerals

Calcium—Calcium is the most abundant mineral in the body and is necessary for many body processes. Patients with inflammatory bowel disease often lack calcium in the diet due to self-limiting of dairy foods such as milk, yogurt, and cheese. In addition to the lack of calcium in the diet, patients exposed to steroids for long durations have an increase in calcium excretion from bone. This side effect can lead to osteoporosis and brittle bones. The RDA for calcium is 800–1200 mg, depending upon need. I always recommend the upper limit of that level.

Body benefits: Calcium is the primary mineral in bones and teeth and accounts for about 39% of the total minerals in the body. Calcium's major function is to maintain the strength of bones and teeth, and approximately 99% of calcium in the body is stored there. Calcium is also responsible for several other bodily functions, such as maintaining normal muscle contraction and relaxation, proper nerve function, blood pressure, blood clotting, and immune defenses.

Deficiencies of calcium are often undetected because blood levels of calcium do not represent levels of calcium in the bone. The presence of osteoporosis may be the first and only sign of calcium insufficiency and may be advanced by the time of detection. Bone density scans may be recommended for IBD patients who have been on steroids often or who have poor calcium intake.

There are many mechanisms by which calcium absorption in the duodenum is increased. These include

- Hormones

- Stomach acid

- Vitamin D

- Lactose

All of these factors favor the absorption of calcium in the body, and that is why a supplement that includes vitamin D is imperative.

Best sources—The body needs calcium every day because absorption occurs on a limited daily basis. Taking massive periodic doses does not help to stabilize calcium in the bone, because the body needs a constant steady rate of absorption. The best sources for calcium in the diet come from low-fat milk products such as milk, cheese, and yogurt. Many IBD patients limit these foods due to intolerance and should therefore compensate with calcium-enriched soy products such as soy milk, soy protein powders with added calcium, soy cheese, and yogurt. Greens are also a good source of calcium; however, greens contain calcium binders called oxalates that make the calcium difficult to absorb. Greens like spinach and broccoli contain a ton of vitamin A; however, they may not be your *body's* best source of calcium.

Iron—Ferrous sulfate, ferrous fumarate, and ferrous gluconate are common forms of this critical mineral. In healthy people, iron is a well-conserved mineral, meaning approximately 90% is re-used. In Crohn's and ulcerative colitis patients, extensive losses from blood and the inability to absorb iron in the duodenum and upper jejunum can cause significant losses of this vital mineral. The rate of iron absorption is under the control of the intestinal mucosa, which if severely damaged has limited capabilities. Other factors that cause problems with iron absorption in IBD include increased transit time of food through the GI tract and fat malabsorption. The RDA for iron is 10 mg for men and post-menopausal women and 15 mg for adolescent and adult females. The needs for IBD patients may be much greater than that depending upon losses. A full blood count is necessary to determine whether or not iron use is warranted, because an excess could lead to excessive storage in the liver.

Body benefits: Iron's main role in the body is to transport oxygen and carbon dioxide in the tissues and lungs. If this critical role is compromised by insufficient supplies of iron, many patients will feel fatigued, confused, and generally weak because of the lack of hemoglobin or oxygen transport to vital organs. Iron also plays a role in cognitive performance, and iron deficiency anemia has been found to decrease mental clarity, learning, and memory in deficient children. Again, I should reiterate that iron can be toxic, and an excess in the body is not to your benefit. A full blood count should be undertaken before starting of any supplement program.

Best sources: The most absorbable form of iron in food is called *heme* iron and is only available in animal protein. Ten to thirty percent of this type of iron can be readily absorbed, whereas only about five percent of iron in vegetables is absorbed. This significant difference in absorption rates makes meat, fish, and poultry the best choices for getting the most absorbable form into the body. Other factors that favor iron absorption include the presence of ascorbic acid, or vitamin C. This antioxidant helps keep the pH of the small intestine higher, which makes iron assimilation much greater. Next time you have some lean-meat protein, grab a small glass of orange juice along with it and you will increase the uptake of iron by about 40%!

Magnesium–I will mention this mineral briefly, because in IBD patients a deficiency can be caused by excess losses due to diarrhea (electrolyte imbalance) and poor absorption from the small intestine. Common manifestations of lack of magnesium include muscle weakness, growth failure, anorexia, and irritability. It is not uncommon to see a deficiency among patients with malabsorption syndromes like IBD. It is difficult to assess a deficiency of magnesium; however, if you have extreme diarrhea you are at greater risk. Diets high in vegetables (especially the kinds that contain chlorophyll), fruits, and unrefined grains tend to be high in magnesium. Meat and dairy are poor sources of this mineral. Also, it should be noted that excess supplementation can lead to more diarrhea; therefore, the best way to stay balanced is to eat more fruits and vegetables containing magnesium and to make sure your multi has a modest amount (about 200mg is sufficient).

Zinc—Zinc is the last of the minerals I will discuss that has relevance to IBD patients. Zinc deficiency occurs most often when there is insufficient intake or when it is poorly absorbed. In IBD, both of those situations are possible, making it important to examine zinc status in the body. Diarrhea greatly increases zinc loss in the body, and when it is significant the need for increasing zinc intake becomes crucial. Deficiency symptoms of zinc often go unnoticed because they can be so pervasive. Growth retardation, hair loss, diarrhea, delayed sexual maturation, and loss of taste sensation and appetite are the most common signs. The RDA for zinc is 11-15 mg/day.

Body benefits—Zinc is critical for various metabolic processes, wound healing, and immune function. We do not fully understand the way the body utilizes zinc, but it is important not to overlook this mineral, because the deficiency symptoms can be severe.

Best sources—The greatest sources of zinc in the diet are red meat, poultry, fortified breakfast cereal, grains, beans, and nuts. Fortification has made getting enough zinc easier; however, a good multivitamin that contains 10–15 mg is also a good idea for IBD patients.

I mention all of these micro-nutrients foremost because they are the most likely deficiencies we see in IBD patients. Quality food choices in the appropriate quantities will help to alleviate many of these inadequacies; however, sometimes food is not enough. Severely poor absorption resulting from a large or small intestine that is incapable of absorbing nutrients needs help beyond what food can supply. Vitamin supplements are one way of getting extra nutrition, but how much you are absorbing still depends upon the functioning of the gastrointestinal tract.

Using calcium as an example, let us look at how the body processes this mineral. Calcium is absorbed mainly in the duodenum and less so in the lower GI tract. If the upper GI tract is damaged, absorption will be compromised more than if only the large intestine is affected. Of all ingested calcium, only 20–30% is absorbed even in healthy individuals. People with less functioning absorptive capabilities may be at only 5–10%. The same is true for the fat-soluble vitamins discussed earlier. Most absorption occurs in the small intestine, and therefore absorption can be very limited by damaged intestinal cells.

In very severe cases of IBD, parenteral nutrition or feeding of nutrients through the bloodstream, may be indicated; however, that is solely reserved for the most extreme cases. Bowel rest through the administration of high-calorie, high-protein liquids may also be reserved for some patients who are intolerant of foods during severe flares. These situations are less common and hopefully never necessary for most IBD patients.

So, how do you get the extra nutrition your body needs beyond food? Look to necessary supplements that give you extra insurance against deficiency and help replace losses. The body may not absorb everything you take in, but by providing extra, you give it a chance to compensate.

Beyond Food—Necessary Supplements

1. *A good multivitamin/multi-mineral formula*

Absorbability counts when it comes to taking vitamins for IBD patients. The easier the dissolution of the vitamin, the more readily it will be assimilated into the body. In other words, form matters. Hard tablets that are not broken down easily may not be as effective as liquids or powder-filled capsules, which are quickly metabolized.

Also of great importance is the content of the multivitamin. Does it have too much vitamin C or magnesium, which can cause excess diarrhea?

Does it provide enough vitamin K and Zinc? I have researched many vitamins and come up with a short list of my favorites:

- Country Life "Multi-Sorb" is a liquid-filled gel capsule that is easy to swallow, contains a balanced amount of micronutrients, and is easily assimilated.

- Lifetime "Softgels" are a similar product with a liquid inside a gel capsule. Again the micronutrient profile is balanced and it is easily absorbed.

- Trace Minerals makes a liquid multivitamin that is quite comprehensive. It is called "Liquimins Liquid Multi Vita-Mineral." It also contains 600 mg of calcium per serving. It is, however, a liquid and may not be palatable to everyone. You can mix it in a little juice if necessary.

- Specifically for children with IBD, there is a liquid multivitamin from Nature's Way that has a good nutritional profile. It is called "Animal Parade" liquid multi for children. They also make a good adult version, called "ReGeneration." The only issue with these vitamins is that they contain about 9 g of sugar per serving.

Taking a high quality multivitamin/multi-mineral supplement is a good way to get a little more nutrient insurance and should be a basic starting place.

2. A highly absorbable calcium supplement (1200 mg—1500 mg as calcium citrate, plus 400 IU vitamin D)

Calcium is a must when it comes to supplements. Even people in the general population should be taking extra calcium to guard against osteoporosis.

For IBD patients, calcium is vital to overall health and should be taken daily. We know that many people with IBD avoid dairy, so taking extra calcium is especially important. The form it comes in deserves a separate explanation, because there are so many to choose from. *According to the National Institutes of Health, the most absorbable form of calcium is the citrate form.* Why? Calcium needs stomach acid to become soluble for the bloodstream to absorb it through the small intestine. As we age, we produce less hydrochloric acid in the stomach, making it more difficult to uptake calcium. Approximately 4% of calcium carbonate is absorbed by people with insufficient stomach acid, whereas the same people will absorb 45% of calcium as citrate form.

Calcium carbonate is a less expensive form of calcium and is less "bulky" than the citrate form. It is suitable in younger people, who produce enough stomach acid, but not for more mature people, above the age of thirty.

Beyond the type of calcium, the form of preparation is important to consider. Hard tablets that contain binding agents can be difficult for even a healthy person to break down. Calcium citrate should be taken as a capsule or liquid. Most tablets are just too hard for the GI tract to break down. These are my recommendations for calcium supplements:

• Lifetime "Liquid Calcium Magnesium" is a complete calcium supplement that contains a good ratio of calcium citrate to magnesium and vitamin D, and it is pre-acidified, making absorption readily accessible to the body. It comes in many flavors, tastes great, and is very easy to take because you just need a spoonful for 600-750 mg. This is a good choice for children or for those who have difficulty swallowing pills.

• Solaray, Twinlab, Country Life, and Nature's Way all make calcium citrate capsules. You may choose the product with vitamin D or not, because the multivitamins recommended already contain this vitamin. Also, some calcium supplements have magnesium and some do not. If the magnesium adds to your diarrhea, choose the calcium citrate capsule that does not include magnesium. One last note: calcium citrate capsules are bulky, and you need to take three to five of them to get the appropriate amount of calcium. This is difficult for many; however, it is a necessity for the prevention of osteoporosis. The liquid may be best for those who do not wish to swallow more pills.

3. Folic acid (800 mcg to 1 mg per day)

The evidence for the benefits of taking folic acid were discussed previously, so it should suffice to say that it is critical to include this dietary supplement in your daily regimen.

I cannot emphasize enough the importance of this B vitamin. If you doubt the magnitude, look up the evidence in the references I have supplied for chapter 5. Take this vitamin in a capsule.

- Solgar makes a tiny easy-to-swallow 800 mcg capsule

- 1 mg dose is by prescription only

4. Probiotics (a high-quality source every day)

There is tremendous research going on in the field of inflammatory bowel disease with regard to bacteria and its causative role in the pathogenesis of Crohn's disease and ulcerative colitis. It is postulated that bacteria in the gut actually causes the over activation of the immune system, which leads to the influx of inflammatory cells that trigger IBD. For this reason, researchers believe that adding beneficial bacteria to the gut can help minimize the effect of "bad" bacteria by keeping the flora in the gut in good balance. More specifically, probiotics help reduce the number of bad bacteria adhering to the intestinal wall, which in turn reduces the number of pro-inflammatory cytokines. Good bacteria like acidophilus, bifidobacterium, and lactobacillus, help to keep more pathogenic bacteria in check.

One important caveat here is that not all probiotics are created equal. Recently, many clinical studies have addressed one specific product that has been proven to help induce remission in ulcerative colitis and chronic pouchitis (inflammation of the pouch after removal of the colon). This evidence has been clearly documented and is supported by many doctors in the field. The name of this product is "VSL#3," and it is available by calling 1-866-get VSL3.

Other high quality products I have used include "Culturelle" and "Healthy Trinity" from Natren. These products are available in the refrigerator section of any good health food store. Both are very high quality in terms of their preparation methods and standards of bacteria per bottle; however, research papers have examined only VSL#3.

5. *Fish oil capsules (a total of 2.7 grams of EPA/DHA per day)*

This supplement is optional but recommended due to clinical data supporting the use of essential fatty acids.

Eating a lot of fish is a great way to get a dose of inflammatory-fighting eicosapentaenoic acid (EPA). However, research indicates that taking a supplement can help even more.

EPA is an omega-3 fatty acid that assists the body in producing "good" prostaglandins. These are chemical messengers that tell the body to reduce the production of "bad" prostaglandins and leukotrienes that increase pro-inflammatory cytokines. This process reduces inflammation and tissue damage within the body.

Numerous studies in prestigious journals including *Journal of Gastroenterology* and the *New England Journal of Medicine* reported that taking 2.7 grams of fish oil capsules every day could reduce the risk of relapse and improve disease symptoms among IBD patients. Specifically, reports indicated that mean disease severity scores declined by as much as 56% among those taking supplements. Also, relapse rates at one year of supplementation were at 28% versus 69% among the control group. That translates into 59% of patients still being in remission after one year of EPA supplements.

It has also been observed that IBD patients have an "abnormal" fatty acid profile in the gut and that this deficiency interferes with the renewal of cells in the intestine. The correction of this deficiency helps the gut repair tissue damage and restore good fatty acid profiles.

The problem with taking fish oil supplements has always been the large quantity of pills needed and the "repeating" taste after taking them. All EPA supplements, however, are not created equal. Freshness and purity levels, in terms of heavy metals, are important overall considerations. I found one product that was superior in quality and exceeded pharmaceutical standards for purity.

This particular product was even used in many clinical trials to determine the efficacy of fish oils. There are probably other products on the market that are good, but Nordic Naturals' "Ultimate Omega" has clinical data backing up its claims. It can be found at *nordicnaturals.com* or 1-800-662-2544.

6. Iron when necessary (amount must be determined by deficiency present).

Iron deficiency is common in IBD, but not everyone needs it to take extra. The best way to determine if an iron deficiency anemia is present is with a simple blood test. If you have a lot of bleeding and you are fatigued and weak, this is a good place to start. Ask your doctor to look at your hemoglobin and hematocrit to determine whether you need this supplement. Iron can be stored in body tissues and an excess can be toxic to the liver, therefore, it is important to determine its necessity.

Iron comes in many forms and all are absorbed quite well. The gentlest form on the stomach is called iron bis-glycinate. There is also ferrous fumarate and ferrous gluconate, which are suitable.

Solgar makes an iron supplement called "gentle iron," which contains the bis-glycinate form.

In Summary

Understanding your disease is the most important aspect to creating wellness in your life. The impact of inflammation can be minor or extensive depending upon the location and the extent of disease.

Crohn's disease that affects the small intestine will lead to the most severe nutritional consequences because of the risk of malabsorption of all micro-and macro-nutrients. Disease in the large intestine can lead to electrolyte imbalances, anemia, and malabsorption of some nutrients due to severe diarrhea. Know where your disease is and the functional capacity of that area of the intestine to best meet your own needs. I have provided you with an overview of why nutrition is essential in all cases of IBD. However, it is important to look within yourself to determine your exact needs.

At the beginning of this chapter, I discussed many nutrients in depth to give you an understanding of the importance of vitamins and minerals. Striving to get most of these critical nutrients from food is your major goal. Food is the best medicine for replacing lost nutrients, and when it is consumed in adequate amounts with the right distribution of nutrients, you will have great success in helping you body heal and feel well. Many times this disease causes severe fatigue and lethargy. It can of course be the inflammation and immune system causing this feeling; however, we must not forget that nutritional deficiencies can also lead to feeling "sick."

When food is not enough, turn to nutritional supplements for extra insurance. All of the recommendations I have made are imperative for IBD patients to meet nutritional challenges in the face of malabsorption. These nutrients will help to minimize deficiencies and cut your risks for nutrition related complications in IBD, especially osteoporosis. Only through education can you free your body of control by this disease. Nutrition can give you the power to control at least this aspect of your health.

In Conclusion

I have walked many miles in the same shoes as you, facing the challenges of this illness—the anxiety, the stress, and the fear of the unknown. Along the way, I have encountered many things that have aided my recovery process and things that have hindered it.

Nutrition, being my passion, has helped to empower my body and mind to be strong. It has given me the courage to control at least one aspect of my disease, re-nourishing my body and allowing my intestines to heal. This has had a tremendous impact on my overall health. However, embracing all modalities toward healing is the true answer to recovery.

Taking time to care for your self physically and emotionally is a necessity in IBD. Nutrition and medication help to heal the body, while hope and faith help to restore the spirit. Having faith in your doctors and your recovery process is paramount to relieving the stress and anxiety that accompany this illness. Having hope in your body's ability to heal itself through all of these means is freedom.

Seek support through family, friends, and local chapters of CCFA. Reduce stress through relaxation, deep breathing, and physical activity. Explore the answers to all of your questions so you can find peace in your life. Coming to terms with this disease is not an easy task; it requires much strength and determination.

My dream in writing this book was to inspire other patients with inflammatory bowel disease to be well. I wanted to encourage people to see that diet and nutrition is an integral part of the healing process and that food is medicine. My hope is that you will use this knowledge and experience to see that the course of this dis-ease can be changed by how you manage your life and *what you eat.*

PART II
Nutrient-Rich Recipes

Fruits and vegetables contain extraordinary compounds called phytochemicals that have been proven to fight cancer and improve the immune system. Several studies have found that people who eat high amounts of fruits and vegetables have one-half the risk of cancer, and less mortality from cancer, than those whose diets were low in fruits and vegetables. It was also found that fruits and vegetables were most effective against cancers that involved epithelial cells, like cancer of the lung, cervix, esophagus, colon, and stomach. Eating well is essential to staying well in healthy individuals and especially in those with chronic disease.

As you go through the recipes in this book, you will find a discussion at the top of each page describing the benefits of eating that particular food. The objective of the recipes is to deliver a significant amount of nutrition in a small quantity of food. What does that mean? It means that most foods I have chosen are high in nutrient density. For example, the butternut squash soup is filled with vitamin A, as beta-carotene, and even a small amount gives you a tremendous amount of nutrition. Throughout the pages, I will discuss other vital nutrients, such as vitamin C, potassium, calcium, folic acid, and all fat-soluble vitamins like A,D, E, and K.

About the recipes...

The recipes in this book are meant to nourish the body while allowing the bowel to be soothed. The combinations of foods provide high concentrations of vitamins and minerals, prepared in a non-irritating manner to support bowel health and reduce inflammation.

You will find that many of the recipes use pureed items, well-cooked vegetables, blended fruits, and high-protein combinations. Maximizing absorption and eliminating stress on the bowel is the goal of these meals.

The simple recipes in this book will give you ideas for breakfast, lunch, and dinner without having to wonder, "is this ok to eat?" Use the principles outlined in this book to be creative with your food choices so you can expand the scope of your diet. Do not be afraid to try foods in different forms (such as pureed soups). You may love them, and the amount of nutrition in one serving is immense. Nourish your body and be open to trying a new way of thinking about food and healing.

Nutrient-Rich Muffins and Super Smoothies

Nutrient-Rich Muffins

Morning Glory Muffins
Pumpkin Spice Muffins
Banana Cinnamon Muffins
Applesauce Muffins with Streusel Topping

Super Smoothies

Vanilla Peach High-Protein Shake
Vanilla Pineapple Banana Shake
"PB" Vanilla Banana Yogurt Shake
Super Mango Smoothie
Cranraspberry Orange Slushy
Chocolate-Covered Banana Shake

Morning Glory Muffins

Morning glory muffins are made with shredded carrots and crushed pineapple. They are moist, delicious, and filled with vitamins. One cup of shredded carrot contains over 40,000 IU of vitamin A. Pineapple has a good amount of potassium and vitamin C. Children love these muffins because they are similar to carrot cake but without the excess fat and sugar. Enjoy them any time of day.

Yields 12 medium-size muffins

¼ cup of canola oil
4 tbs. melted butter
½ cup brown sugar
1 cup shredded carrots
½ cup crushed pineapple
¾ cup of milk
¼ cup of yogurt
2 large eggs
1 tsp. vanilla
2 cups all-purpose flour
½ tsp. baking powder
1 tsp baking soda
1 tsp. cinnamon
¼ tsp ginger

Heat oven to 350° F and spray two six-count muffin pans with Pam.

Mix first nine ingredients in a large bowl and whisk together.

In a separate bowl, mix all dry ingredients and then add them to the wet mixture being careful not to over-mix the batter. Stir just until all ingredients are incorporated.

Spoon batter into pans and top with cinnamon sugar. Bake for 20–25 minutes or until golden brown on top.

Pumpkin Spice Muffins

Imagine getting half your daily requirement for vitamin A in one small muffin. Unbelievably rich in carotenoids, pumpkin is a sure winner when it comes to adding nutritive value to your food. One cup of canned pumpkin yields 54,040 IU of that powerhouse nutrient to your breakfast. Forget the usual pancakes or waffles; muffins can be low in fat and sugar and be rich in vitamins if you use the proper ingredients. They are also easy to eat on the run!

Yields 12 medium-size muffins

¼ cup canola oil
4 tbs. melted butter
¼ cup packed brown sugar
¼ cup sugar
1 cup lactose-free milk
1 cup canned pumpkin
2 large eggs
1 tsp vanilla
2 cups flour
2 tsp. baking powder
½ tsp. baking soda
1 tsp. cinnamon
1 tsp. pumpkin pie spice
¼ tsp salt
Cinnamon sugar for topping

Heat oven to 350° F and spray two six-count muffin tins with Pam.

Mix first eight ingredients in a large bowl and whisk together.

In a separate bowl, mix all dry ingredients and then add them to the wet mixture, being careful not to over-mix the batter. Stir just until all ingredients are incorporated.

Spoon batter into pans and top with cinnamon sugar. Bake for 20 minutes or until golden brown on top.

Banana Cinnamon Muffins

These muffins are moist and flavorful and are a good source of potassium and soluble fiber. Soluble fiber slows digestion and potassium is an electrolyte that is often lost during a flare-up. Try these muffins for a snack or for breakfast. The yogurt in the recipe contributes only a small amount of lactose, because yogurt is naturally fermented.

Yields 12 medium muffins

¼ cup canola oil
4 tbs. melted butter
½ cup brown sugar
¹/₃ cup plain yogurt
¾ cup lactose-free milk
2 large eggs
1 tsp. vanilla
1 cup all-purpose flour
1 cup oat flour
½ tsp. baking powder
½ tsp. baking soda
1 tsp. cinnamon
¼ tsp salt
2 large ripe bananas diced small

Heat oven to 375° F and spray two six-count muffin tins with Pam.

Mix first seven ingredients together in a large bowl and use a whisk to incorporate some air into the batter.

In a separate bowl, blend the dry ingredients and then add them to the wet mixture. Stir just enough to combine all ingredients being careful not to over-mix the batter. Lastly, add the diced banana and fold in gently.

Place batter in muffin tins three-quarters of the way to the top and bake for 20–22 minutes.

Applesauce Muffins with Streusel Topping

These muffins are a great way to start your day. Packed with soluble fiber from the applesauce and oat flour, these muffins help to slow things down in your gut. Remember, soluble fiber helps the intestine absorb water, whereas insoluble fiber speeds things up. Easy to eat and super tasty, these "soft" fiber muffins will soon become a favorite.

Yields 12 medium size muffins

¼ cup canola oil
4 tbs. melted butter
½ cup packed brown sugar
1¼ cup unsweetened applesauce or apricot applesauce
2 large eggs
1 tsp vanilla
1½ cups all-purpose flour
½ cup oat flour
2 tsp. baking powder
¼ tsp. salt
1 tsp cinnamon
½ tsp. pumpkin pie spice

Heat oven to 400° F and spray two six-count muffin tins with Pam.

Mix first six ingredients in a large bowl and whisk together.

In a separate bowl, combine all dry ingredients and then fold the mixture into the wet ingredients. Do not over-mix; stir only until combined.

Make the topping:

> 4 tbs. softened butter
> ½ cup flour

¼ cup sugar

½ tsp cinnamon

With clean hands, mix butter with other ingredients in a small bowl, using your fingers to cut the butter in and form a crumbly mixture.

Pour muffin batter into tins and top with the streusel mix. Bake for 25 minutes.

Vanilla Peach High-Protein Shake

*Adding a protein powder to a shake gives you a lot of extra protein and vita-
mins. I like to use a soy powder called Spiru-tein.*

*Spiru-tein adds 14 grams of protein to this shake, as well as the equivalent
of a multivitamin and 30% of the daily value for calcium. With the addition
of milk, one shake has 22 grams of protein and 60% of the daily value for calcium. This is a great meal-replacement shake, and I often use it when my
appetite is poor.*

Serves 1

1 scoop vanilla Spiru-tein
1 cup of lactose-free milk or soy milk
4 slices frozen peaches
¼ cup orange juice
Ice

*Mix all ingredients in an ice crushing blender or smoothie maker. Serve imme-
diately.*

Vanilla Pineapple Banana Shake

Once again add a soy protein powder to this shake for extra nutrition. The vanilla has a nice mild flavor that pairs well with banana and pineapple. The addition of these fruits contributes a good amount of potassium which is great for those with chronic diarrhea. This shake also has 22 grams of protein and 60 % of the daily value for calcium.

Serves 1

1 scoop vanilla Spiru-tein
1 cup lactose-free milk or soy milk
½ of a frozen banana
¼ cup of pineapple juice
Ice

Mix all ingredients in an ice crushing blender or smoothie maker. Serve immediately.

"PB" Vanilla Banana Yogurt Shake

Many IBD patients are lactose intolerant; however, yogurt is not the same as milk. Since yogurt is a fermented product, the lactose is already broken down into its component sugars, glucose and galactose. For this reason, high quality yogurt, like Fage (Greek yogurt), Erivan, and Stonyfield, which do not have added milk solids, are well tolerated. This is a great breakfast shake due to the beneficial bacteria content, potassium, and calcium. The peanut butter also adds great flavor, texture, and calories.

Serves 1

1 cup soy milk or lactose-free milk
1 scoop vanilla Spiru-tein
½ cup plain or vanilla yogurt
½ banana
1 tbs. smooth peanut butter
Crushed ice

Mix all ingredients together in an ice-crushing blender or smoothie maker. Serve immediately

Super Mango Smoothie

Smoothies are great for breakfast or to have as an afternoon snack. This version is packed with 40% of the daily value for calcium and is also rich in vitamins and minerals from the mango and orange juice. Mango and orange juice together are full of vitamin A and potassium. Enjoy this smoothie for a great pick-me-up.

Serves 1

1 cup soy milk or lactose-free milk
½ cup calcium-fortified orange juice
5 chunks frozen mango
½ banana
Crushed ice

Mix all ingredients in an ice-crushing blender or smoothie blender. Serve immediately

Note: *I prefer to use soy milk over regular milk when possible. Soy is rich in isoflavones and does not promote mucous production, as milk does. Try Silk vanilla soy milk in this recipe. You will never know the difference, and the calcium content is the same as milk.*

Frozen mango can be purchased in the frozen section at your supermarket or health food store.

CranRaspberry Orange Slushy

This is a refreshing warm weather drink that provides a nutritious alternative to the typical sugar-laden commercial slushy drinks.

Using fruit juice combined with frozen banana provides over 100% of the RDA for vitamin C along with 20% of the RDA for calcium and a good amount of potassium. Enjoy this drink at snack time or for dessert.

Serves 1

6 oz. calcium-fortified orange juice
4 oz. cranberry-raspberry cocktail
4 chunks frozen banana
½ cup crushed ice

Mix all ingredients in an ice-crushing blender or smoothie maker and serve immediately.

Chocolate-Covered Banana Shake

Sometimes people with IBD are bothered by chocolate. I like to use a chocolate flavored protein powder that does have some cocoa but does not seem to cause any GI distress. This is a great shake to have in the afternoon when chocolate cravings creep up. Add some frozen banana for potassium and good nutritive value.

Serves 1

1 cup soy milk or lactose-free milk
1 scoop Spiru-tein chocolate soy powder
4–5 chunks of frozen banana
Crushed ice

Mix all ingredients in an ice-crushing blender or smoothie maker. Serve immediately.

Sustaining Soups and Salads

Sustaining Soups

Sweet Butternut Squash and Apple Soup
Old-Fashioned Chicken Noodle Soup
Harvest Vegetable Soup
Tomato Rice Soup
Sweet Potato and Carrot Soup
Gingered Carrot with Honey Soup
Escarole, Carrot, and Potato Soup
Pastina with Spinach and Carrot Soup
Potato and Carrot Soup
Egg Drop Soup with Spinach

Salads

Boston Lettuce Salad with Artichoke Hearts and Roasted Peppers
Avocado and Roasted Red Pepper Salad with Cilantro Vinaigrette

Sweet Butternut Squash and Apple Soup

Butternut squash is extremely rich in nutrients. One cup yields 7290 IU of vitamin A and 896 mg of potassium. The recommended dietary allowance for vitamin A is 5000 IU, so one bowl of this soup packs a nutritious punch. The cooked apple provides bowel slowing soluble fiber.

Serves 6

½ of an onion, chopped
2 tbs. butter
2 tbs. canola oil
6 cups butternut squash, peeled and cut (2 large; *supermarkets usually have this available already peeled and cut)*
2 apples, peeled and cubed
48 oz.of homemade or store-bought chicken or vegetable broth
3 tbs. honey
Salt and pepper to taste

In a large soup pot, sauté onion in butter and oil until soft. Add squash and apple and cook for 5 minutes. Add broth to the pot and bring to a boil. When soup is boiling, lower heat and simmer for 45 minutes.

Turn off heat once vegetables are soft and allow the soup to cool a little. Process the soup in batches using a blender or food processor, placing the pureed soup in a large bowl. Add honey, salt, and pepper to pureed soup. Stir well and serve.

* If you need to gain weight, you may add ½ cup of heavy cream to the pureed soup. Heavy cream has virtually no lactose, because it has a very high percentage of fat. This will add 410 calories to the soup.

Old-Fashioned Chicken Noodle Soup

Everyone loves a bowl of hearty chicken soup, and this is one of the best you will ever make. Made with fresh chicken, carrots, turnips, and noodles, it is a great meal by itself. The carrots and parsnips add quality vitamins, while the chicken gives you high-quality protein and the noodles add some carbohydrate. Serve it the next day for the best flavor.

Serves 6

1 medium onion cut into 4 large pieces
2 celery stalks cut into 4 large pieces
2 tbs. olive oil
1 whole chicken
64 oz. chicken broth
3 cups water

Wash chicken well and remove insides. In a large soup pot, heat olive oil and add onion and celery to pot. Cook vegetables for 3 minutes and then add chicken, broth, and water to the pot. Cover and cook 1 hour.

1 bag baby carrots
2 parsnips peeled
½ pound capellini pasta
Salt and pepper

In a food processor, process the carrots and parsnips with the metal blade until they are chopped into tiny pieces. Add the vegetables to the soup and cook for 30 minutes.

Remove chicken from pot and allow it to cool a bit. Also, remove large chunks of celery and onion, as they are difficult to digest.

Add pasta, salt and pepper to soup and cook 10 more minutes. Remove meat from chicken and add it back to the soup. Serve with a little Parmesan cheese. Enjoy!

Harvest Vegetable Soup

Parsnips, carrots, squash, and potato make this soup rich in vitamins as well as delicious. Make it for fall meals or holidays at home. The rich orange color of the soup tells you it is full of beta carotene and other antioxidants like vitamin C. Getting in your daily veggies is easy, because this soup is a snap to make and it tastes so good!

Serves 6

2 tbs. olive oil
2 tbs. butter
1 small onion, chopped
2 parsnips, peeled and cut
1 butternut squash, peeled and cut
1 16 oz. bag of baby carrots
1 white potato, peeled and cut
32 oz. vegetable or chicken broth
2 cups apple cider
3 tbs. brown sugar
1 tsp. salt, pepper to taste
½ cup heavy cream

In a large soup pot, sauté onion in oil and butter.

When onion is soft, add all vegetables to the pot and cook for 5 minutes. Add broth and cider and continue to cook for 45 minutes, at a simmer.

Remove soup from heat and allow it to cool a little. Place soup in a food processor or blender to puree. Transfer soup to a large bowl and add salt, pepper, and brown sugar.

Pour cream into a small bowl and then put a few tablespoons of soup in to temper the cream (this helps the cream not to curdle). Pour the mixture back into the soup and serve.

Tomato Rice Soup

Cooked tomatoes are one of the greatest sources of lycopene. What is lycopene? Lycopene is a carotenoid that has been proven to reduce the risk of several different cancers, including cancers of the digestive tract and prostate. Lycopene is also a powerful antioxidant that protects the body's cells from free radicals that cause degenerative diseases like atherosclerosis. Prepare this soup often—it is as delicious as it is healthy.

Serves 6

1 medium onion, chopped
1 garlic clove, sliced in two
2 tbs. olive oil
2 tbs. butter
2 28 oz. cans whole tomatoes
3 cups chicken broth
Salt and pepper
1½ cups cooked white rice

In a large soup pot, sauté onion and garlic in oil and butter and cook over low heat.

When onion is translucent, pour tomatoes into the pot along with the broth. Bring soup to a low boil, lower heat, and cook for 45 minutes.

Remove soup from the heat and allow it to cool enough to place contents in a food mill. This will puree the tomatoes and remove the seeds from the soup. Once pureed, place soup into a large bowl and add salt, pepper, and rice.

Serve with a little Parmesan cheese on top.

***Note:** if you do not want to add rice, you may serve this soup with large seasoned croutons. I like to use a crispy Italian bread sliced thin and topped with* *a little olive oil and Parmesan cheese, which I bake in the oven at 400°F for 10 minutes.*

Sweet Potato and Carrot Soup

Two powerhouse vegetables cooked together yields one extremely nutritious soup, filled with vitamin A (as beta carotene) and easily digestible. One sweet potato has approximately 24,750 IU of vitamin A. (Remember, the daily requirement is about 5000 IU.) Add the carrots in and that is a big dose of healthful soup!

Serves 4

2 tbs. butter
2 tbs. olive oil
½ onion diced
1 large sweet potato peeled and diced
2 16 oz. bags of baby carrots
48 oz. chicken broth or vegetable broth
2 tbs. brown sugar
Salt and pepper to taste

In a large soup pot, sauté onion in butter and oil until very soft. Add cut sweet potato and carrots to the pot and stir for 2 minutes.

Add chicken broth and bring to a boil. Reduce heat and allow soup simmer for 45 minutes.

Add brown sugar, salt, and pepper. Remove from heat and allow soup to cool a little before processing in a blender or food processor until smooth.

Gingered Carrot with Honey Soup

Carrots are very high in vitamin A, and 1 cup yields 38,300 IU of this super antioxidant (as beta-carotene). That equals seven times the recommended daily allowance for this powerhouse nutrient.

The ginger in the soup helps to ease digestion and adds great flavor.

Serves 6

½ onion, chopped
2 tbs. butter
2 tbs. canola oil
2 tsp. fresh grated ginger
2 16 oz. bags of baby carrots
48 oz. of chicken or vegetable broth
2 tbs. honey
Salt and pepper to taste

In a large soup pot, sauté the onion in butter and oil. Grate the ginger and add it to the pot, being very careful not to burn it. Add carrots and stir to coat with ginger, about 2 minutes.

Add broth to pot and bring to a boil. Lower heat and cook soup for about 45 minutes or until carrots are soft.

Allow soup to cool a little and then puree it in a blender or food processor. Transfer each batch of pureed soup to a large bowl. When complete, add honey, salt, and pepper to season.

* You may also wish to add ½ cup of heavy cream to this recipe if weight gain is desired. It must be added at the very end to prevent the cream from curdling.

Escarole, Carrot, and Potato Soup

This is a chunky soup that works great as a meal. Escarole is similar to spinach in consistency and is easy on the digestive system. I love to make soups, because even when you cook the vegetables so soft you get all the nutrition, since you are eating the broth they are cooked in. Use Yukon gold potatoes for this recipe—they are sweet and delicious.

Serves 6

½ onion, diced
2 tbs. olive oil
2 whole garlic cloves
4 large carrots, peeled and diced
2 Yukon Gold potatoes, peeled and diced
1 head of fresh escarole
48 oz. chicken broth
1 14 oz. can tomato sauce
Salt and pepper

Prepare all the vegetables for the soup and put aside. The escarole should be washed well and cut into small pieces.

In a large soup pot, heat oil and add onion and garlic. Sauté for a few minutes and then add potato and carrot. Cook over moderate heat for 5 minutes. Add broth and tomato sauce and cook for 30 minutes at a simmer.

When vegetables are tender, add escarole, salt, and pepper. Continue to cook 15 more minutes and serve. Add some good Parmesan cheese for additional flavor.

Pastina with Spinach and Carrot Soup

This is one of the easiest soups to make, and children love it. Pastina is made from egg, so it has a little more protein than regular pasta. When you add in spinach and carrots for vitamin A, you have a meal within itself.

Serves 4

2 tbs. butter
2 tbs. olive oil
4 carrots, peeled and diced
1 package frozen chopped spinach
1 48 oz. can chicken broth
1 cup pastina
Salt and pepper to taste

Sauté chopped carrots in butter and oil for 2 minutes. Add broth to pot and bring to a boil.

Add pastina and stir for 1 minute. Thaw spinach and add to soup, allowing the pasta and spinach to cook at the same time. Continue cooking over medium heat for 10 minutes.

Add salt and pepper and serve.

* Some grated cheese makes a tasty addition when serving. Hard cheeses like Parmesan and Romano are virtually lactose free because they are aged.

Potato and Carrot Soup

This hearty and thick soup is reminiscent of very smooth mashed potatoes. The carrots give it a little color and sweetness. Potato is naturally rich in vitamin C, providing 26 mg in one medium-size potato. The recommended dietary allowance for vitamin C is 90 mg for adults. The carrots add nutritious value to the soup by providing a good amount of beta-carotene.

Serves 4

3 tbs. butter
2 tbs. olive oil
½ onion, diced
3 large Yukon gold potatoes, peeled and diced
1 16 oz. bag baby carrots
48 oz vegetable broth
1 cup lactose-free milk
Salt and pepper to taste

In a large soup pot heat butter and oil until melted. Stir in onion, potato, and carrot and cook for 3 minutes.

Add broth to the pot and bring to a boil. Allow the soup to cook for 45 minutes or until vegetables are very soft.

Cool soup slightly and process in a food processor until smooth. Transfer the soup to a large bowl and then add tempered* milk. Add salt and pepper to taste.

Note**Temper milk by adding a little warm soup to the milk and then pour the mixture into the pureed soup.*

Egg Drop Soup with Spinach

Egg drop soup is one of the simplest soups to prepare and is quite nutritious. Eggs are filled with iron, lecithin, and B vitamins for energy. When you add spinach to the mix, you get a good amount of vitamin A as well. Children love this soup for the taste, and you will love it for the nutrition.

Serves 4

48 oz. chicken broth
4 large eggs
¼ cup lactose-free milk
1 16 oz. bag baby spinach leaves
Salt and pepper

In a large soup pot, heat the broth to a low boil. In a medium sized bowl, mix eggs with milk until scrambled.

Slowly drizzle egg mixture into boiling broth. Allow it to cook for 2–3 minutes and then add washed spinach leaves.

Season with salt and pepper and serve with a little grated cheese if desired.

Boston Lettuce Salad with Artichoke Hearts and Roasted Peppers

You should avoid any lettuce when diarrhea is significant. This salad is accept-able for IBD patients, because the lettuce is very soft and the artichoke hearts and roasted peppers are cooked. Try this as a side dish or a lunchtime meal.

Serves 2

1 head Boston lettuce, washed and cut
1 jar marinated artichoke hearts
2–3 roasted peppers, sliced thin

Combine salad ingredients on a plate and assemble neatly. Top with vinai-grette dressing, recipe to follow.

Vinaigrette:

3 tbs. red wine vinegar
1 tsp Dijon mustard
½ tsp. Salt
2 tbs. olive oil

Whisk together and serve over salad.

Avocado and Roasted Red Pepper Salad with Cilantro Vinaigrette

Why make a salad out of avocado and red peppers? Avocado is one of the richest sources of potassium, a critical electrolyte that helps the body maintain water balance and that is often compromised during episodes of chronic diarrhea.

Red peppers are a highly concentrated form of vitamin C, which helps your immune system fight infection.

Serves 4

1 large haas avocado, sliced
2 large red bell peppers, roasted and peeled, or 1 jar of high-quality roasted peppers

To roast the peppers, place washed peppers under the broiler, turning until each side is blackened. This will take about 5 minutes per side.

Place roasted peppers in a brown bag to steam for 15 minutes and then peel and slice them.

Place avocado slices on a flat plate and top with peppers and dressing. Recipe to follow.

For the dressing;

1 handful fresh cilantro
Juice of 1 lime
2 tbs. white wine vinegar
4 tbs. good olive oil
½ tsp. salt
Pepper to taste

Chop cilantro finely and place in a bowl. Add lime juice and vinegar and whisk together.

Slowly stream in olive oil while whisking mixture together. This will allow the dressing to emulsify. Whisk in salt and pepper and serve over salad.

Meat Entrees

Chicken

Roasted Chicken with Lemon and Herbs
Chicken with Spinach and Shitake Mushrooms
Chicken with Pasta, Spinach, and Roasted Peppers in Marsala Wine Sauce
Grilled Chicken Sandwiches with Pesto Mayonnaise and Roasted Peppers
Thai Chicken with Jasmine Rice

Pork

Center-Cut Pork Chops with Apricot Glaze
Pork Tenderloin with Homemade Applesauce

Red Meat

Stuffed Red Peppers
Savory Beef Stew with Wine and Vegetables

Roasted Chicken with Lemon and Herbs

When all else fails, chicken is a safe bet. This dish is very traditional and hearty, and it provides a good source of lean protein. Serve this dish with roasted root vegetables, as they work well together.

Serves 4

2 bone-in chicken breasts, split
Juice of 1 lemon
3 tbs. olive oil
2 sprigs fresh rosemary
3 tbs. fresh thyme, chopped
3 tbs. fresh sage, chopped
2 garlic cloves, sliced in half
Salt and pepper to taste

Wash the chicken and leave the skin on.

Place the chicken in a roasting pan and drizzle it with olive oil. Squeeze lemon juice on top and sprinkle on all the herbs. Place garlic in the pan and then season chicken with salt and pepper.

Roast chicken at 375°F for about 1 hour. When eating the meat, remove the skin. Cooking it with the skin allows the chicken to stay moist.

Chicken with Spinach and Shitake Mushrooms

This is a great way to serve chicken, even to guests. This dish combines lean protein with highly nutritious greens and shitake mushrooms. Many of the Chinese mushrooms, like shitake and maitake, are noted for their cancer-fighting benefits. Some people even choose to take them in supplement form; however, I prefer to use them fresh.

Serves 4

1 pound chicken breast, pounded into filets ¼-inch thin
½ cup flour
Salt and pepper
1 large bag of washed spinach, stems removed
1 garlic clove, sliced into three pieces
1 tbs. olive oil
3 tbs. butter
3 tbs. olive oil
1 cup chicken broth
¾ cup white wine
8 shitake mushrooms, washed and sliced with stems removed

Dredge chicken in flour that is seasoned with salt and pepper and set aside.

In a large sauté pan, warm garlic in olive oil and quickly wilt the spinach season with a little salt and pepper.

Remove spinach from pan and place it in a serving platter. Add butter and olive oil to pan and brown chicken slightly on both sides. Add broth and cook chicken covered for 10 minutes.

Add mushrooms and wine and continue cooking for 5–7 more minutes. Place chicken and mushrooms on top of spinach and enjoy! You may add a little more salt and pepper if needed.

Chicken with Pasta, Spinach, and Roasted Peppers in Marsala Wine Sauce

This dish is very tasty and combines ingredients that are filled with great nutrition. The spinach is a great source of the carotenoids, beta-carotene, and lutein, as well as folic acid. The roasted red peppers add a good amount of vitamin C to the dish. Chicken provides lean protein, and pasta gives you some complex carbohydrate for energy!

Serves 6

Flour for dredging
Salt and pepper
1 pound boneless skinless chicken breast
¼ cup butter (½ stick)
2 tbs. olive oil
1 large jar roasted red peppers
¾ cup Marsala wine
1 cup chicken broth
4 cups washed fresh spinach leaves
1 pound cooked penne pasta

Cut chicken into cubes and dredge in flour seasoned with salt and pepper.

In a large sauté pan, heat butter and oil. Place chicken in pan and brown on all sides, about 10 minutes.

Cut peppers into strips and add to chicken. Immediately add chicken broth and wine. Cook for 5 minutes.

Add spinach and a little more salt and pepper. Cook until spinach is just wilted and pour over hot pasta.

Grilled Chicken Sandwiches with Pesto Mayonnaise & Roasted Peppers

These sandwiches are great on the grill for a summertime meal. The pesto mayonnaise adds a lot of flavor without the traditional additions of garlic and pine nuts, which can cause GI upset. Add the roasted peppers for color and nutrition. They are rich in antioxidants and flavor.

Serves 4

Pesto Mayonnaise:

> 1 large handful fresh basil
> Juice of 1 lemon
> ¼ cup mayonnaise
> 2 tbs. Parmesan cheese

Chop basil finely, place in a bowl with all other ingredients, and refrigerate until ready to serve.

Chicken:

> 1 pound boneless chicken breast
> 2 tbs. olive oil
> 2 tbs. rice wine vinegar
> Juice of 1 lemon
> 1 tsp. Italian seasoning
> Salt and pepper
> 1 jar roasted peppers or fresh

Marinate chicken in the above ingredients for 1 hour. Grill chicken for 15–20 minutes, depending upon thickness.

Place cooked chicken on non-seeded rolls with pesto mayonnaise and top with roasted peppers.

Note: if you are one of those who can tolerate cheese other than the hard ones, try some Asiago or fresh mozzarella on top.

Thai Chicken with Jasmine Rice

This extremely flavorful dish is scented with fresh ginger and cilantro. The peanut butter and tamari help to make a thick and tasty sauce for the chicken. Jasmine rice is a nice accompaniment, and it can usually be found in your regular supermarket.

Serves 4

3 tbs. smooth peanut butter
3 tbs. tamari (dark soy sauce)
3 tbs. rice wine vinegar
¼ cup apple juice
2 tsp. honey
Juice of 1 lime
4 tbs. canola oil
1 tsp. grated fresh ginger
Handful of fresh cilantro, chopped
1 pound chicken breast, cut into cubes

Mix first six ingredients together in a blender, slowly drizzle in canola oil, and add ginger and cilantro. Pour marinade over prepared chicken and place in the refrigerator to marinate for 2–3 hours.

Pour chicken and marinade into a large sauté pan and cook over medium heat covered for 15 minutes. Stir in between to cook all sides of the chicken.

Prepare jasmine rice according to directions and serve chicken on top. Garnish with a squeeze of lime and a little extra chopped cilantro.

Center-Cut Pork Chops with Apricot Glaze

Center-cut pork chops are among the leanest meats you can eat. Not only is white meat pork lean, but it is also one of the most outstanding food sources of the B vitamin thiamin. Thiamin is important for energy metabolism and overall health of the nervous system.

Serves 4

1 pound boneless center-cut pork chops (4 chops 1" thick)
Salt and pepper
2 tbs. olive oil
1 tbs. Dijon mustard
$^1/_3$ cup apricot preserves
3 tbs. balsamic vinegar

Wash and dry pork chops and season with salt and pepper.

In a large skillet, brown chops on both sides in olive oil. Remove them from the pan, leaving the drippings.

While the pan is still hot, add balsamic vinegar and reduce it for 2 minutes. Add mustard and preserves to the pan and whisk together.

Place pork chops back in pan and continue to cook them covered over low heat for 15 minutes, or until an internal thermometer reads 165°F. Serve chops on a platter topped with sauce.

Pork Tenderloin with Homemade Applesauce

Pork tenderloin is one of the leanest meats you can eat. It has about 2 grams of fat per 1-ounce serving, making it leaner than white-meat chicken. Pork is also very high in the B vitamin thiamin, which is an important part of energy metabolism. The applesauce is an important addition to the meal for its content of soluble fiber, which helps to slow the bowel.

Serves 4

1 pound pork tenderloin
Salt and pepper
½ cup low-sodium soy sauce
3 tbs. rice wine vinegar
2 tbs. sesame oil
2 tbs. honey
1 tbs. grated fresh ginger
½ cup pineapple juice

Unwrap tenderloin, wash it, salt and pepper the outside, and put it in a 13 × 9 pan to marinate.

Prepare marinade in a saucepan, adding all remaining ingredients to pot and cooking over low heat for 5 minutes.

Allow marinade to cool and pour over tenderloin. Refrigerate meat for 2–3 hours, covered.

Cook meat on a grill or in the oven at 375 degrees to an internal temperature of 165° F, about 30 minutes.

Slice meat into 1" slices and serve with homemade applesauce, recipe to follow.

Homemade Applesauce

Homemade applesauce is an easy treat to prepare and is great as a snack or as part of the meal above.

Serves 4

3 Mackintosh apples, peeled and diced
1 Granny Smith apple, peeled and diced
2 tbs. brown sugar

In a medium-size pot, add all ingredients and cook over low heat, covered for about 20 minutes. Cover should be tight to allow steam to stay in the pot.

Once apples are very soft, put the mixture in a food mill or food processor to puree. Leave applesauce a little chunky if you prefer it that way.

Stuffed Red Peppers

Use red peppers in this recipe for their antioxidant value and sweet flavor. One red bell pepper has the nutrient value of a full day's requirement of vitamins A and C. Imagine getting all that nutrition at one meal!

When stuffing the peppers, I use lean chopped meats to provide good protein and rice to slow the bowel. These are great for dinner or lunch and are quite easy to make.

Serves 4

For the stuffing:

> 1 pound top-quality mixed chopped meat (turkey, pork, beef)
> 2 cups of cooked white rice
> ½ tsp. Salt
> Black pepper
> $^1/_3$ cup Parmesan cheese
> 6 oz. tomato sauce (1 small can)

Cook the meat over moderate heat in oil until fully browned. Add cooked rice, salt, pepper, Parmesan, and tomato sauce. Heat through for 5 more minutes. Remove from heat.

For the peppers:

> 4 large red bell peppers
> 16 oz. tomato sauce
> Salt and pepper
> Sprinkling of Parmesan cheese

Wash the peppers well, slice off tops, and clean seeds out of the middle. Place peppers standing up in a shallow baking dish. A 13 × 9 pan works well to secure the peppers.

Place stuffing in each pepper and fill to the top. Pour tomato sauce in the bottom of the pan and over the peppers. Give peppers a sprinkling of salt, pepper, and Parmesan cheese.

Bake covered with tin foil at 375° F for 30 minutes. Remove foil and cook for 10 more minutes or until peppers are very soft.

When eating, peel the skin off. This should be easy to do, and it will help you digest the peppers more easily.

Savory Beef Stew with Wine and Vegetables

I am not a big advocate for eating a lot of red meat; however, once a month is acceptable. Beef does have the most absorbable form of iron, called "heme iron"; therefore, it is especially suitable for those who are anemic. The long cooking process, along with the wine, breaks down the meat's collagen, allowing it to become very tender. Add the veggies for a great one-pot meal.

1 pound stew meat
Flour for dredging
Salt and pepper
2 tbs. olive oil
½ onion, chopped
1 garlic clove, sliced in half
12 oz. beef broth
½ cup red wine Pinot Noir works well
1 can diced tomatoes
2 tbs. ketchup
2 tbs. Worcestershire sauce
1 16 oz. bag of baby carrots
2 potatoes, peeled and diced
½ tsp. salt
Pepper to taste

Dredge meat in flour salt and pepper.

In a large stew pot, heat the oil. Place meat into pot and brown lightly on all sides on high heat.

Lower heat to medium and add onion and garlic slices.
Once meat is fully browned and onion is soft (6–7 minutes), add broth, wine, tomatoes, ketchup, and Worcestershire.

Bring mixture to a boil and reduce heat to a low simmer allowing the stew to cook for approximately 1 hour.

After one hour, add carrots and potatoes and cook 1 hour longer.
Add salt and pepper and enjoy!

Fabulous Fish

Shrimp Franchase
Shrimp with Asparagus in Wine Sauce
Breaded Baked Lemon Sole
Grey Sole Stuffed with Spinach
Salmon with Honey Mustard
Salmon with Lemon Zest and Herbs
Swordfish with Cilantro Mayonnaise
Swordfish with Mango Pineapple Salsa
Tilapia Buerre Blanc
Tuna Steak Teriyaki

Shrimp Franchase

By combining two lean proteins, you get a lot of value out of one meal. Shrimp is easy to digest and low in fat. Eggs provide the benefit of iron, B vitamins, and lecithin. Enjoy this meal paired with herbed rice and spinach for a well-rounded dinner.

Serves 4

1½ pounds cleaned tail-on jumbo shrimp
½ cup flour, seasoned with salt and pepper
3 eggs, beaten
3 tbs. butter
2 tbs. olive oil
2 lemons
½ cup white wine
Fresh parsley
Salt and pepper to taste

Dip shrimp in flour and egg and set aside. Heat a large skillet and melt butter and olive oil together.

Add shrimp to pan and brown slightly on both sides (about 2 minutes each side). Squeeze juice from 1½ lemons into pan and then add wine and parsley.

Continue to cook for about 5 minutes, add a little more salt and pepper, and serve immediately.

Garnish with other ½ of lemon.

Shrimp with Asparagus in Wine Sauce

Shrimp is a very lean protein that happens to be easily digested and well liked by most. When you pair it with asparagus, you add a lot in the way of vitamins, especially folic acid. Folic acid is one of the most important B vitamins in protecting our cells and preventing DNA damage to them.

Serve this dish over rice to complete the meal. Everyone in the family will enjoy it.

Serves 4

1½ pounds cleaned jumbo shrimp
½ cup flour
Salt and pepper
5 tbs. butter
2 tbs. olive oil
Juice of 1 lemon
½ cup chicken broth
1 pound asparagus, washed and cut into 2" pieces
½ cup good white wine
Salt and pepper

Dredge shrimp in flour seasoned with salt and pepper and set aside.

In a large sauté pan, cook shrimp in butter and oil for about 3 minutes. Add lemon, broth, and asparagus and cook covered over medium heat for 4 more minutes.

Add wine, salt, and pepper and cook uncovered for 2 more minutes. Serve immediately over rice.

Breaded Baked Lemon Sole

Believe it or not, children just love fish prepared this way. It reminds them of breaded chicken and yet they get the benefits of fish.

Fish of any kind can give you a good amount of lean protein and is easily digested. You don't always have to eat oily fish, although it does have the highest content of essential fatty acids. When you need a change, try some shellfish or white fish.

Serves 4

1 pound lemon sole
Salt and pepper
2 cups seasoned breadcrumbs
2 large eggs
3 tbs. olive oil
Lemon for garnish

Wash fish, sprinkle with salt and pepper, and dip pieces in egg.

Next, dip fish in breadcrumb mixture and place on baking sheet with the olive oil. Bake at 375° F for about 20 minutes.

Grey Sole Stuffed with Spinach

I use Grey sole in this recipe because it is very sweet and not the least bit fishy. You may choose to use lemon sole if that is all you can find. This dish has a good amount of lean protein from the fish (35 grams per 5 oz. serving), and when you combine that with the spinach for vitamins and minerals, you have a great one-dish meal.

Serves 4

For the stuffing:

> ½ of an onion, diced fine
> 2 tbs. olive oil
> 1 box frozen chopped spinach, thawed
> 3 tbs. high-quality Parmesan cheese (like Parmigiano Reggiano)
> ½ cup bread crumbs
> ½ tsp. salt, pepper to taste

Prepare the stuffing in a large skillet by first sautéing the onion in olive oil until very soft. Next add the spinach, cheese, and breadcrumbs and cook for 5 minutes.

For the fish:

> 1 pound fresh Grey sole
> Salt and pepper
> Paprika
> Lemon juice from one lemon
> 2 tbs. butter

Wash fish and put salt and pepper on both sides.

Lay each filet flat and put ½ cup of stuffing in center. Fold ends over and place rolled filet end down on a shallow baking pan.

Top fish with paprika for color, sprinkle with lemon juice, and dab each piece with a teaspoon of butter. Bake at 375° F for 20 minutes.

Salmon with Honey Mustard

Salmon tastes great with the flavors of honey and mustard. This dish is easily prepared and is packed with inflammation-fighting omega-3 fish oils. Try to use wild salmon when available to reduce the risk of toxin exposure. Farmed salmon has been questioned lately for its content of PCBs.

Serves 2

1 pound wild salmon (1" thick)
2 tbs. Dijon mustard
2 tbs. honey
Salt and pepper

Wash salmon and place it in a baking pan. Season with salt and pepper and set aside.

Mix mustard with honey and place it on top of salmon.

Bake at 375° F for 20 minutes.

Salmon with Lemon Zest and Herbs

It's not always easy making fish tasty when you are limiting garlic and strong spices. This dish has great flavor and the benefit of a high content of omega-3 fatty acids. Remember, these essential fatty acids help the body to reduce inflammation. Several research studies have proven this fact, and although supplements may also help, eating fish at least two times a week is a must. When choosing salmon, ask for wild salmon over farmed.

Serves 4

2 large handfuls of fresh dill
1 large lemon
1 tbs. Dijon mustard
½ tsp. pressed garlic
3 tbs. good extra-virgin olive oil
Salt and pepper to taste
1½ pounds fresh wild salmon
Salt and pepper

For the topping, wash dill and lemon, and with a large chef's knife, finely chop dill and add 2 tbs. zest from the lemon.

Transfer to a bowl and add juice from the lemon, mustard, and garlic.

Slowly drizzle in a fine stream of olive oil while whisking; this will help to emulsify the topping.

Wash fish and top with salt and pepper. Transfer to a baking pan with sides and top with herb mixture. Allow to marinate covered, in the refrigerator, for 1 hour.

Cook at 375° F for 20–25 minutes. You may also cook this on your grill, using a disposable tin lasagna pan and cooking covered for 20–25 minutes.

Swordfish with Cilantro Mayonnaise

Swordfish is one of those oily fish that has the benefit of omega-3 fatty acids, which help to reduce inflammation.

Try to get this fish fresh, as the frozen varieties are sometimes rubbery and less appealing. Any fish should be eaten three times per week, and this is a very flavorful dish to try one of those days.

Serves 2

2 handfuls fresh cilantro, chopped finely
¼ cup mayonnaise
Juice of one whole lemon
Salt and fresh pepper
1 pound fresh swordfish
1 tablespoon olive oil
Juice of 1 lemon
Salt and fresh pepper

Put the first four ingredients in a food processor (or just mix by hand) and put aside.

Wash the fish, place it in shallow baking dish, drizzle with olive oil and lemon, and season with salt and pepper.

Heat oven to 375° F and cook fish for 10 minutes. Top with cilantro sauce and finish cooking for another 10–15 minutes, depending on the thickness of the fish. Serve immediately.

Note: you may choose to grill the fish. Follow the same method, but cooking time may be shorter.

Swordfish with Mango Pineapple Salsa

Recently there has been much controversy over the Mercury content of sword-fish. Although some of the information may be troubling I still believe the ben-efits of eating these oily fish outweigh the negatives associated with it. Swordfish provides a good amount of omega 3 fatty acids to the diet. These essential fatty acids help the body fight inflammation and help to improve any inflammatory process. Add some mango to this dish for great flavor and vitamins.

Serves 4

Marinade

2 tbs. olive oil
Juice of 1 lime
Salt and pepper
1½ pounds fresh swordfish

Salsa:

> 1 fresh mango peeled and diced
> ½ cup pineapple diced
> 1 handful fresh cilantro leaves chopped fine
> 2 tbs. canola oil
> 2 tbs. lime juice
> 1 tbs. rice wine vinegar
> Salt and pepper to taste

Wash fish and sprinkle both sides with salt and pepper.

Combine olive oil and lime juice and dress fish with this marinade. Allow to marinate in the refrigerator for 1 hour.

Mix remaining ingredients together for salsa and allow salsa flavors to combine for at least one hour. (This may stay at room temperature.)

Cook swordfish on the grill or in a pan for about 10 minutes per side for a 1"-thick piece. Cook longer, if necessary, until fully done on the inside. (It should be white.)

Top with salsa and serve immediately.

Tilapia Buerre Blanc

Tilapia has a very mild flavor and a light, flaky texture. Tilapia is not a very oily fish, but it is still a great source of lean protein and is easy to find fresh or frozen. This dish is simple and can be prepared in about 15 minutes. Buerre is French for butter, and blanc *means white so I have used white wine.*

Serves 2

Flour for dredging
Salt and pepper
1 pound tilapia
2 tbs. butter
1 tbs. olive oil
1 garlic clove, sliced
Juice of 1 lemon
¼ cup white wine
6–7 fresh basil leaves

Wash and dry fish and dredge in flour that seasoned with salt and pepper.

In a large sauté pan, heat butter and oil and add garlic. Cook garlic until soft but not brown.

Add fish to pan and cook on both sides until slightly browned, about 4 minutes on each side.

When browned, add lemon and wine to pan and cook down 4 more minutes. Add fresh basil and a little more salt and pepper, if desired.

Tuna Steak Teriyaki

Tuna steak is a good source of omega-3 fatty acids, those essential fats that help the body fight inflammation. This method of preparation is very simple and flavorful. I allow the fish to marinate for at least 4 hours so it can become very full flavored. Tuna is usually served rare, but I do not recommend serving it this way for IBD patients. Your fish should always be cooked through to ensure the least risk of bacterial contamination.

Serves 2

1 pound sushi-grade tuna steak
3 tbs. canola oil
3 tbs. soy sauce
1 tbs. fresh grated ginger
¼ cup pineapple juice, plus 4 pineapple rings
2 tbs. duck sauce or apricot jam
Juice of ½ a lemon

Wash tuna steak and set aside in a marinating dish.

In a medium-size bowl, mix all marinade ingredients, setting aside pineapple slices, and pour over fish. Cover and refrigerate for 4 hours.

To cook fish on the grill, sear both sides for 3 minutes and then continue cooking over medium heat for 15 more minutes or until fully cooked. (Twenty minutes per inch of thickness is a good rule.)

To serve marinade with the fish, you must cook it first. Bring marinade to a boil and allow it to cook at a simmer for 10 minutes. Serve with pineapple slices on top.

Vegetables and Other Side Dishes

Vegetable Side Dishes

Butternut Squash and Carrot Puree
Braised Swiss Chard
Sautéed Spinach
Roasted Winter Vegetables with Rosemary
Roasted Asparagus

Other Side Dishes

Egg and Spinach Frittata
Pasta with Fresh Tomato Sauce
Pasta with Broccoli
"Fried" Rice with Carrots and Shitake Mushrooms
Spinach and Rice

Butternut Squash and Carrot Puree

This is a great side dish for autumn or winter meals or for holiday gatherings. The rich orange color tells you powerful antioxidants are at work in these vegetables. As discussed in several other recipes, butternut squash and carrot are filled with beta-carotene, a pro-vitamin A carotenoid that helps support the body in many critical ways.

Serves 4

1 large butternut squash, peeled and cubed
1 16 oz. bag baby carrots
4 tbs. butter
¼ cup brown sugar
Salt and pepper

In a large soup pot, add enough water just to cover vegetables and cook for about 30 minutes or until very tender.

Drain vegetables with a strainer and place them in a food processor fitted with a metal blade.

Add butter and brown sugar while still hot. Puree until very smooth and add salt and pepper to taste.

Braised Swiss Chard

To braise means to cook with liquid, which in this case makes the Swiss chard very soft. Swiss chard is one of those forgotten vegetable that is actually quite delicious and healthful. Similar in quality to spinach, Swiss chard is loaded with vitamin A as beta-carotene and is easy to digest. Use this as a side to a protein-rich meal.

Serves 4

1 large head of Swiss chard
2 garlic cloves, sliced in half
2 tbs. olive oil
¾ cup chicken broth
Salt and pepper

Wash chard and cut into large pieces.

Heat olive oil in a sauté pan and cook garlic over low heat for 5–7 minutes. Throw in chard and sauté 2 minutes.

Pour in chicken stock and cover, allowing chard to cook for 10 minutes. Remove lid and allow some of the liquid to evaporate. Season with salt and pepper to taste.

Sautéed Spinach

Pound for pound, spinach is one of the most nutritious vegetable you can eat. The only vegetable that might top it is kale. One cup of cooked spinach gives you 245 mg of calcium, 839 mg of potassium, and 14,742 IU of vitamin A. Spinach is easy on the digestive system, as long as it is cooked, and is great as a side dish to any meal.

Serves 4

1 large bag of baby spinach
1 clove of fresh garlic
1 tbs. olive oil
1 tbs. butter
Salt and pepper

Wash spinach very well and remove any tough stems. The baby spinach should not have much stem, but regular spinach will.

Cut garlic into three slices. In a medium-size sauté pan, cook garlic over low heat in oil and butter—do not brown the garlic at all.

When garlic is soft (6 minutes), add spinach to pan and cook over moderate heat for 5 minutes. Add salt and pepper to taste.

Note: cook with garlic in large pieces and then remove it from your food. You will get the benefit of flavor without the detrimental digestive effects.

Roasted Winter Vegetables with Rosemary

It is hard to find vegetables that patients with IBD can tolerate, and many just avoid them altogether. I like to be creative when preparing food, and this dish combines many root vegetables that have a lot of vitamin A (as beta-carotene) and great flavor. The high-heat cooking method makes these vegetables soft and easily digested.

Serves 4

1 pound carrots, peeled and cut into 2" pieces
2 parsnips, peeled and cut into 2" pieces
1 turnip, peeled and cut into 2" pieces
½ butternut squash, peeled and cubed
2 tbs. olive oil
2 tbs. butter
Salt and pepper
3 fresh rosemary sprigs

Place all vegetables except squash in oil, butter, salt, pepper, and rosemary in a large roasting pan.

Heat oven to 450°F and roast vegetables for 20 minutes.

Add squash and continue to cook for 25 more minutes. Serve as a side dish to roasted chicken.

Roasted Asparagus

Asparagus are extremely healthful but often overlooked when it comes to vegetables. Asparagus are filled with vitamin K, important for blood clotting, and folate, critical for DNA synthesis, cancer prevention, and the prevention of birth defects.

Besides all these great health benefits, asparagus are easily digested and are a snap to prepare. Try this 10-minute recipe.

Serves 4

1 pound fresh asparagus
2 tbs. olive oil
Salt and pepper
¼ cup breadcrumbs
2 tbs. good Parmesan cheese

Wash asparagus and trim bottoms about 3 inches.

Heat oven to 450° F and place asparagus on a baking pan. Season with salt, pepper, and 1 tbs. olive oil.

Toss breadcrumbs with remaining olive oil and cheese and top asparagus. Place in oven for 10 minutes to roast and serve immediately.

Egg and Spinach Frittata

Eggs are a great source of protein, iron, B vitamins, and lecithin. Most people only think of eating eggs in the morning. Try this for lunch or dinner as a highly nutritious creation that is easily prepared and acts as a one-dish meal because of its high nutrient content.

Serves 4

1 tbs. butter
1 tbs. canola oil
2 cups fresh baby spinach
5 large eggs
1/3 cup lactose free milk
Salt and pepper
3 tbs. Parmesan cheese

In a large nonstick skillet, melt butter with oil and sauté spinach until wilted.

Beat eggs with salt, pepper, and milk, and add to pan. Cook over medium heat, lifting the sides of the egg as it cooks to allow the liquid on top to get to the bottom of the pan.

Cook for about 7–8 minutes and top with Parmesan cheese.

Remove from heat and cover for 3 minutes. Eggs should be fully cooked with no liquid on top. Serve immediately.

Pasta with Fresh Tomato Sauce

Tomatoes are one of the greatest sources of the carotenoid lycopene, so I like to use them quite often. The seeds of the tomato can be troublesome, so you must strain this sauce with a food mill or fine strainer to remove them. The pasta in this dish provides necessary carbohydrate and calories.

Serves 6

1 medium onion
2 garlic cloves
3 tbs. extra-virgin olive oil
2 cans plum tomatoes
2 teaspoons sugar
2 teaspoons salt
Black pepper
6–8 fresh basil leaves

Peel onion and cut in quarters. Peel garlic and slice in half. In a large soup pot, heat the olive oil over low heat and add onion and garlic.

Sauté onion and garlic until softened, about 10 minutes, being careful not to burn the garlic. Meanwhile, puree the tomatoes in a blender and then strain them to remove the seeds.

Add tomato to pot and allow mixture to cook for 30 minutes.

Add sugar, salt, and pepper. Cook 15 more minutes and then add basil. Use sauce to top cooked pasta and serve with a little good Parmesan cheese.

Note: The sauce will have large pieces of garlic and onion. These are used to flavor the sauce but should not be eaten by IBD patients as they may cause distress. Take them out of the sauce or just avoid them.

Pasta with Broccoli

Cruciferous vegetables like broccoli contain phytonutrients, such as sulforaphane and dithiolthiones. These compounds have been studied recently for their ability to trigger enzymes that block carcinogenic damage to cells.

Broccoli, kale, and other greens are extremely healthy to eat but can be somewhat troublesome for IBD patients. This recipe allows the broccoli to cook for a long time in broth to soften the fiber matrix. Although this helps in digestion, broccoli still causes gas and should be eaten only when diarrhea is not severe.

Serves 4

2 tbs. extra-virgin olive oil
1 garlic clove, sliced
48 oz. chicken broth
1 large head broccoli, cut in florets
1 pound penne pasta
Salt and pepper to taste

In a large soup pot, sauté garlic over low heat in olive oil.

Add chicken broth and heat to a simmer. Wash broccoli and add it to the pot. Bring mixture to a full boil.

Add pasta to pot and cook for 10–12 minutes more. Season with salt and pepper and serve with good quality Parmesan cheese.

"Fried" Rice with Carrots and Shitake Mushrooms

This is a great side dish that pairs well with the teriyaki tuna. It is also nutritious due to the vitamin A in the carrots and the powerful medicinal properties in the shitake mushrooms. The rice provides some complex carbohydrate and helps to slow things down in the gut.

Serves 4

2 large carrots
10 shitake mushrooms
¼ cup soy sauce
2 tbs. canola oil
1 tbs. butter
2 large eggs
2 cups cooked white rice
Salt and pepper, if needed

Peel the carrots and cut them into small, thin rounds. Cook the carrots in boiling water until soft. Drain and set aside.

Wash the mushrooms well, remove the stems, and slice thin.

Heat a large nonstick skillet and cook the mushrooms in oil and butter, sautéing, them for about 5 minutes.

Place the rice in the pan with the mushrooms and stir constantly, allowing the rice to get a little brown. Put soy sauce in and push the rice to one side of the pan.

Toss eggs in on the other side of the pan and scramble them a bit before mixing them with the rice mixture.

Mix carrots in and continue cooking for about 5 more minutes until the "fried" rice is well mixed and has a nice golden color.

* Hint: Sometimes I use leftover rice for this dish; even if the rice is a little dry, this dish brings it back to life.

Spinach and Rice

I like to combine spinach with rice because at times the spinach may move through the GI tract too quickly. The rice helps to slow things down and makes diarrhea less likely. Spinach is, of course, one of the most nutritious vegetables we can eat, so try this as a side dish to a meal that contains some form of good-quality protein, such as fish or chicken.

Serves 4

1 14 oz. can chicken broth
1 tbs. butter
1 cup white rice
1 package frozen chopped spinach
2 tbs. olive oil
Salt and pepper to taste

Cook rice according to directions on the package and substitute the broth for water.

Microwave the spinach and add olive oil, salt, and pepper.

Add spinach to fully cooked rice and heat through for 3 more minutes. Serve immediately.

Three Quick Desserts

Banana Cream Pie
Peach Crisp
Baked Apples with Cinnamon

Banana Cream Pie

What could be better tasting than banana cream pie with a dollop of cream? Banana cream pie may not sound too healthy, and I will not say it is, but as far as desserts go it does have some advantages over your typical piece of cake. The milk in the pudding provides a bit of calcium, and the banana provides potassium. You can choose to make this pie without added sugar by using a "no added sugar" pudding mix.

Serves 6

2 large bananas, peeled and sliced
1 box vanilla pudding mix
2 cups lactose-free milk
1 ready graham crust
Non-dairy whipped topping

Place sliced banana in bottom of piecrust and set aside.

Mix pudding according to directions and pour over bananas. Place pie in refrigerator for at least one hour and serve with a dollop of whipped topping.

Peach Crisp

As I stated earlier when discussing desserts, it is important to eat a dessert that has some value beyond taste. Fruit desserts are satisfying ways to cure cravings, and they have some nutritious value. Peaches, for example, have a bit of potassium and vitamin A. This fruit crisp also has oatmeal in the topping for a healthy crunch and some soluble fiber. Fruit crisps use less sucrose (white sugar) than many other desserts, because the fruit is sweet enough.

Serves 6

6 large, slightly soft peaches
¼ cup light brown sugar
Juice of one lemon
1 teaspoon cinnamon

Wash and peel peaches then cut them into long 1" slices. Place peaches in an 8 × 8 baking pan and toss with sugar, lemon, and cinnamon. Set aside.

For the topping:

       ½ cup all-purpose flour
       ½ cup oatmeal
       ¼ cup white sugar
       ¼ cup light brown sugar
       2 tsp. Cinnamon
       ½ cup butter

Mix flour, oatmeal, sugars, and cinnamon in a bowl.

Cut butter into tiny pieces and, using your fingers, mix butter into flour mixture. Keep mixing butter in with your fingers until a crumbly texture is achieved.

Place crumb mixture on top of peaches and bake at 350° F for 45 minutes.

Baked Apples with Cinnamon

I have never been a great fan of eating a lot of sugar and I believe that when it comes to dessert, it is best to choose one with some value. Here is the last of the three desserts that have some value beyond taste. They have a bit of nutrition—from the fruit! Remember, the inside of the apple provides a good amount of soft soluble fiber when baked. This helps slow down the bowel.

Serves 4

4 large Rome apples, peeled
4 tsp. cinnamon
4 tbs. reduced sugar maple syrup
½ cup 7-Up

Place peeled apples in an 8 × 8 inch baking dish and top each apple with 1 teaspoon of cinnamon and 1 tablespoon maple syrup.

Pour 7-Up into the bottom of the pan to moisten the apples and keep the pan from burning.

Bake the apples uncovered at 350° F for 1 hour. Serve warm and enjoy!

References

Chapter One: Who This Book is Written For

Janowitz, Henry D. *Your Gut Feelings.* New York: Oxford University Press,1989.

Reinhard, Tonia. *Gastrointestinal Disorders and Nutrition.* New York: McGraw Hill Companies, 2002.

Scala, James. *The New Eating Right for a Bad Gut.* New York: Penguin Putnam Inc, 2000.

Mahan, L., Kathleen and S. Escott-Stump. *Krause's Food Nutrition and Diet Therapy.* Philadelphia: Saunders, 1999, 2000.

Shils, M. E., J. A. Olson, and M. Shike. *Modern Nutrition in Health and Disease.* Philadelphia: Lea and Febiger, 1994.

The Crohn's and Colitis Foundation of America. Library: Diet, Nutrition, and Fitness. *Available at: <<hhp://www.CCFA.org/medicalcentral/ library/diet/eat.htm>>* [accessed date March 2005].

Chapter Two: The Eight Principles of Eating Well with Inflammatory Bowel Disease

Campos, F. G. "Inflammatory Bowel Diseases. Principles of Nutrition Therapy." *Rev. Hosp. Clin. Med. S. Paulo* 57(4)(2002): 187-198.

Jeejeebhoy, R. N. "Clinical Nutrition: Management of Nutritional Problems of Patients with Crohn's Disease." *Canadian Medical Association Journal* 166(7)(2002): 913-923.

Badart-Smook A. R.; W. Stockbrugger; R. J. Brummer; B. J. Geerling. "Comprehensive Nutritional Status in Recently Diagnosed Patients with Inflammatory Bowel Disease Compared with Population Controls." *European Journal Clinical Nutrition* 54(6): (2000)514-521.

Motil, K. J.; R.J. Grand; L Davis-Kraft; L.L. Ferlic; E. D. Smith. "Growth Failure in Children with Inflammatory Bowel Disease: A Prospective Study." *Gastroenterology* 105(1993) : 681-691.

Pearson, M.; K.Teahon; A. J. Levi; I. Bjarnoson. "Food Intolerance and Crohn's Disease." *Gut* 34(1993): 783-787.

Ferguson, A.; M. Glen; and S. Ghosh. "Crohn's Disease: Nutrition and Nutrition Therapy." *Baillieres Clin. Gastroenterology* 12(1)(1998): 93-114.

Ballegaard, M.; A. Bjergstrom; S. Brondum; et al. "Self-Reported Food Intolerance in Chronic Inflammatory Bowel Disease." *Scand. Journal of Gastroenterology* 32(6)(1997): 569-571.

Colditz, G. A.; L. G. Branch; R.J. Lipnic. "Increased Green and Yellow Vegetables Intake and Lowered Cancer Death in an Elderly Population." *American Journal of Clinical Nutrition* 41(1985): 32-36.

Joachim, Gloria. "Responses of People with Inflammatory Bowel Disease to Food Consumed." *Gastroenterology Nursing* 23(4)(2000): 160-167.

Mishkin, S. "Dairy Sensitivity, Lactose Malabsorption and Elimination Diets in Inflammatory Bowel Disease." *American Journal of Clinical Nutrition* 65(1997): 564-567.

Jeejeebhoy, K. N. "The Many Faces of Malnutrition in Crohn Disease." *American Journal of Clinical Nutrition* 67(1998): 819-820. (editorial).

Imes, S.; B. R. Pinchbeck; A. B. R. Thomson. "Diet Counseling Modifies Nutrient Intake of Patients with Crohn's Disease." *Journal of the American Dietetic Association* 87(1987): 457-462.

Pennington, Jean A., and Judith Douglass. *Bowes and Church's Food Values of Portions Commonly Used, 18th ed.* Philadelphia: J. B. Lippincott, Williams & Wilkins, 2005.

Mahan, L., Kathleen and Marian Arlin. *Krause's Food Nutrition and Diet Therapy, 8th ed.* Philadelpia: Saunders, 1999, 2000.

Recommended Dietary Allowances, 10th ed. Washington, D. C.: National Academy Press, 1989.

Shils, M. E., J. A. Olson, and M. Shike. *Modern Nutrition in Health and Disease, 8th ed.* Philadelphia: Lea and Febiger, 1994.

Whitney, Eleanor, C. Cataldo, S. Rolfes. *Understanding Normal and Clinical Nutrition, 3rd ed.* New York: West Publishing, 1991.

The Crohn's and Colitis Foundation of America. Library: Diet, Nutrition, and Fitness. *Available at:* <<hhp://www.CCFA.org/medicalcentral/library/diet/eat.htm>>.

National Institutes of Health. Office of Dietary Supplements. Dietary Supplement Factsheets for Vitamin A., Vitamin D, Magnesium, Calcium, Iron and Zinc. Bethesda, Maryland, 2004.

Chapter Three: Food Safety

Bunning, V. K.; J. A. Lindsay; and D. L. Archer. "Chronic Health Effects of Microbial Foodborne Disease." *World Health Stat.* 50(1-2)(1997): 51-56.

Lindsay, James A. "Chronic Sequelae of Foodborne Illness." *Emerging Infectious Disease* 3(4)(1997): 1-12.

Applied Foodservice Sanitation: A Certification Coursebook, 4th ed.

The Educational Foundation of the National Restaurant Association, 1992.

Bcan, N. H.; J. S. Goulding; C. Lao; and F. J. Angulo. "Surveillance for Foodborne Disease Outbreaks." *United States, CDC Surveillance Summary* 45(1996): 1-66.

Websites: Humans as Hosts of Foodborne Disease *<<IFT.org/IFT/ Research/expertreports/microfilm—report.htm>>* [accessed December, 2005}

Chapter Five: The Need for Vitamins and Minerals and When to Supplement

Geerling, B. J.; R. W. Stockbrugger; and R. J. M. Brummer. "Nutrition and Inflammatory Bowel Disease. An Update." *Scand. Journal Gastroenterol* 34(1999): 95-105.

Han, P. D.; A. Burke; R. N. Baldassano; et al. "Nutrition and Inflammatory Bowel Disease." *Gastroenterol Clin.* 28(1999): 423-436.

Jeejeebhoy, K. N. "Clinical Nutrition: 6. Management of Nutritional Problems of Patient's with Crohn's Disease." *Canadian Medical Association Journal* 166(7) (2002): 913-923.

Institute of Medicine. Food and Nutrition Board. Dietary Reference Intakes for Vitamin A, Vitamin K, Arsenic, Boron, Chromium, Copper, Iodine, Manganese, Molybedeum, Nickel, Silicon, Vanadium, and Zinc. Washington, DC: *National Academy Press,* 2001.

National Institutes of Health. Office of Dietary Supplements. Dietary Supplement Factsheets for Vitamin A, Vitamin D, Magnesium, Calcium, Iron and Zinc. Bethesda, Maryland, 2004.

Kampman, E.; M. Slattery; C. Bette; J. Potter. "Calcium, Vitamin D, Sunshine Exposure, Dairy Products and Colon Cancer Risk." *Cancer Causes Control* 11(2000): 459-466.

Tsujikawar, Tomoyuki, et al. "Clinical Importance of N-3 Fatty Acid-rich Diet and Nutritional Education for the Maintenance of Remission in Crohn's Disease." *Journal of Gastroenterology* 35(2000): 99-104.

Belluzzi, Andrea, et al. "Effect of an Enteric Coated Fish Oil Preparation on Relapses in Crohn's Disease." *The New England Journal of Medicine* 334(1996): 1557-1560.

Siguel, Edward, and Robert H. Lerman. "Prevalence of Essential Fatty Acid Deficiency in Patients with Chronic Gastrointestinal Disorders." *Metabolism* 45(1996): 12-23.

Aslan, Alex and George Tridafilopoulos. "Fish Oil Fatty Acid Supplementation in Active Ulcerative Colitis: A Double-blind Placebo Controlled, Crossover Study." *American Journal of Gastroenterology* 87(1992): 432-437.

Joachim, G. "The Relationship Between Habits of Food Consumption and Reported Reactions to Food in People with Inflammatory Bowel Disease—Testing the Limits." *Nutr. Health* 13(2) (1999): 69-83.

Shanhan, F. "Probiotics and Inflammatory Bowel Disease: Is There a Scientific Rationale?" *Inflammatory Bowel Disease* 6(2) (2000):107-115. Review.

D. A. Zhong Cao, et al. "Effects of Folic Acid on Epithelial Apoptosis and Expression of Bcl—2 and P 53 in Pre-Malignant Gastric Lesions." *World Journal of Gastroenterology* 11(2005): 1571-1576.

Freudenheim, J. L.; S. Graham; J. R. Marshall; B. P. Haighey; S Cholewinski; G. Wilkinson. "Folate Intake and Carcinogenesis of the Colon and Rectum." *Int. Journal Epidemiology* 20(1991): 368-374.

Carrier, J., et al. "Effects of Dietary Folate on Ulcerative Colitis-Associated Colorectal Carcinogenesis in the Interleulein—2 and Beta (2) Microglobulin—Deficient Mice." *Cancer Epidemiol Biomarkers Prev.* 12(2003): 1262-1267.

Lashner, B. A. "Red Blood Cell Folate is Associated with the Development of Dysplasia and Cancer in Ulcerative Colitis." *J. Cancer Res. Clin. Oncol.* 119(9) (1993): 549-554.

Lashner, B. A.; P. A. Heidenreich; G. L. Su; S. V. Kane; S. B. Hanover. "Effect of Folate Supplementation on the Incidence of Dysplasia and Cancer in Chronic Ulcerative Colitis. A Case-Control Study." *Gastroenterology* 97(2) (1989): 255-9.

Geerling, B. J.; A. Badart-Smook; R. W. Stockbrugger; R. J. Brummer. "Comprehensive Nutritional Status in Recently Diagnosed Patients with Inflammatory Bowel Disease Compared with Population Controls." *Eur. J. Clin. Nutr.* 54(6) (2000): 514-521.

Han, P. D.; A. Burke; R. N. Baldassano; J. L. Rombeau; G. R. Lichtenstein. "Nutrition and Inflammatory Bowel Disease." *Gastroenterology Clin. North America* 28(2) (1999): 423-443.

Capristo, Esmeralda, et al. "Nutritional Status and Energy Metabolism in Crohn's Disease." *The American Journal of Clinical Nutrition* 69(2) (1999): 339-340.

Craig, Winston. Phylochemicals: Guardians of our Health. Vegetarian Nutrition. *Available at:* <<hhp://www.andrews.edu/NUFS/phyto.html>> [accessed May 1, 2005].

The Crohn's and Colitis Foundation of America. Library: Diet, Nutrition, and Fitness. *Available at:* <<hhp://www.CCFA.org/medicalcentral/library/diet/eat.htm>> [accessed March,2005].

Schoon, E. J.; M. C. Muller; C. Vermeer; L. J. Schurgers; R. J. Brummer; R. W. Stockbrugger. "Low Serum and Bone Vitamin K Status in Patients with Longstanding Crohn's Disease: Another Pathogenetic

Factor of Osteoporosis in Crohn's Disease?" *Gvt.* 48(4) (2001): 473-477.

Bibiloni, Rodrigo; R. N. Fedorak; Gerald, Tannock; et al. "VSL #3. Probiotic Mixture Induces Remission in Patients with Active Ulcerative Colitis." *The American Journal of Gastroenterology* 100(7) (2005): 1539-1572.

Dotan, I. and D. Rachmilewitz. "Probiotics in Inflammatory Bowel Disease: Possible Mechanisms of Action." *Current Opinions Gastroenterology* 21(4) (2005): 426-430.

Fedorak, R. N. and K. L. Madsen. "Probiotics and the Management of Inflammatory Bowel Disease." *Inflammatory Bowel Disease* 10(3) (2004): 286-299.

Sartor, R. B. "Therapeutic Manipulation of the Enteric Microflora in Inflammatory Bowel Diseases: Antibiotics, Probiotics, and Prebiotics (abstract)." *Gastroenterology* 126(6)(2004): 1620-1633.

Pennington, Jean A., and Judith Douglass. *Bowes and Church's Food Values of Portions Commonly Used, 18th ed.* Philadelphia: J. B. Lippincott, Williams & Wilkins, 2005.

Mahan, L., Kathleen and Marian Arlin. *Krause's Food Nutrition and Diet Therapy, 8th ed.* Philadelpia: Saunders, 1999, 2000.

Recommended Dietary Allowances, 10th ed. Washington, D. C.: National Academy Press, 1989.

Shils, M. E., J. A. Olson, and M.Shike. *Modern Nutrition in Health and Disease, 8th ed.* Philadelphia: Lea and Febiger, 1994.

Whitney, Eleanor, C. Cataldo, S. Rolfes. *Understanding Normal and Clinical Nutrition, 3rd ed.* New York: West Publishing, 1991.

The Crohn's and Colitis Foundation of America. Library: Diet, Nutrition, and Fitness. *Available at: <<hhp://www.CCFA.org/medicalcentral/library/diet/eat.htm>>.*

National Institutes of Health. Office of Dietary Supplements. Dietary Supplement Factsheets for Vitamin A., Vitamin D, Magnesium, Calcium, Iron and Zinc. Bethesda, Maryland, 2004.

978-0-595-39749-5
0-595-39749-2